COMPACT Research

Leukemia

Diseases and Disorders

ReferencePoint Press®

San Diego, CA

Select* books in the Compact Research series include:

Current Issues

Abortion
Animal Experimentation
Biomedical Ethics
Cloning
Conflict in the Middle East
The Death Penalty
Energy Alternatives
Free Speech
Genetic Engineering
Global Warming and Climate Change
Gun Control
Illegal Immigration
Islam
Media Violence
National Security
Nuclear Weapons and Security
Obesity
School Violence
Stem Cells
Terrorist Attacks
U.S. Border Control
Video Games
World Energy Crisis

Diseases and Disorders

ADHD
Alzheimer's Disease
Anorexia
Autism
Bipolar Disorders
Hepatitis
HPV
Meningitis
Phobias
Sexually Transmitted Diseases

Drugs

Alcohol
Antidepressants
Club Drugs
Cocaine and Crack
Hallucinogens
Heroin
Inhalants
Marijuana
Methamphetamine
Nicotine and Tobacco
Performance-Enhancing Drugs
Prescription Drugs
Steroids

Energy and the Environment

Biofuels
Deforestation
Hydrogen Power
Solar Power
Wind Power

*For a complete list of titles please visit www.referencepointpress.com.

COMPACT Research

Leukemia

by Peggy J. Parks

Diseases and Disorders

ReferencePoint Press®

San Diego, CA

ReferencePoint Press®

For more information, contact:
ReferencePoint Press, Inc.
PO Box 27779
San Diego, CA 92198
www. ReferencePointPress.com

Picture credits:
Cover: iStockphoto.com
Maury Aaseng: 32–35, 47–49, 61–63, 75–77
Science Photo Library: 12, 17

LIBRARY OF CONGRESS CATALOGING-IN-PUBLICATION DATA

Parks, Peggy J., 1951–
Leukemia / by Peggy J. Parks.
p. cm. — (Compact research series)
Includes bibliographical references and index.
ISBN-13: 978-1-60152-099-9 (hardback : alk. paper)
ISBN-10: 1-60152-099-9 (hardback : alk. paper)
1. Leukemia—Juvenile literature. I. Title.
RC643.P355 2009
616.99'419—dc22

2009029702

Contents

Foreword

“Where is the knowledge we have lost in information?”

—T.S. Eliot, “The Rock.”

As modern civilization continues to evolve, its ability to create, store, distribute, and access information expands exponentially. The explosion of information from all media continues to increase at a phenomenal rate. By 2020 some experts predict the worldwide information base will double every 73 days. While access to diverse sources of information and perspectives is paramount to any democratic society, information alone cannot help people gain knowledge and understanding. Information must be organized and presented clearly and succinctly in order to be understood. The challenge in the digital age becomes not the creation of information, but how best to sort, organize, enhance, and present information.

ReferencePoint Press developed the *Compact Research* series with this challenge of the information age in mind. More than any other subject area today, researching current issues can yield vast, diverse, and unqualified information that can be intimidating and overwhelming for even the most advanced and motivated researcher. The *Compact Research* series offers a compact, relevant, intelligent, and conveniently organized collection of information covering a variety of current topics ranging from illegal immigration and deforestation to diseases such as anorexia and meningitis.

The series focuses on three types of information: objective single-author narratives, opinion-based primary source quotations, and facts and statistics. The clearly written objective narratives provide context and reliable background information. Primary source quotes are carefully selected and cited, exposing the reader to differing points of view. And facts and statistics sections aid the reader in evaluating perspectives. Presenting these key types of information creates a richer, more balanced learning experience.

For better understanding and convenience, the series enhances information by organizing it into narrower topics and adding design features that make it easy for a reader to identify desired content. For example, in *Compact Research: Illegal Immigration*, a chapter covering the economic impact of illegal immigration has an objective narrative explaining the various ways the economy is impacted, a balanced section of numerous primary source quotes on the topic, followed by facts and full-color illustrations to encourage evaluation of contrasting perspectives.

The ancient Roman philosopher Lucius Annaeus Seneca wrote, "It is quality rather than quantity that matters." More than just a collection of content, the *Compact Research* series is simply committed to creating, finding, organizing, and presenting the most relevant and appropriate amount of information on a current topic in a user-friendly style that invites, intrigues, and fosters understanding.

Leukemia at a Glance

What Leukemia Is

Leukemia is a cancer of the blood that is characterized by an overproduction of abnormal white blood cells (or leukocytes), which flood the bloodstream, crowd out healthy cells, and prevent normal cell death from happening.

Types of Leukemia

Leukemia is classified according to the type of cell that is affected and whether the disease is acute (fast growing) or chronic (slow growing). The four most common types are acute myeloid (or myelogenous) leukemia, chronic myeloid leukemia, acute lymphocytic leukemia, and chronic lymphocytic leukemia.

Prevalence

More than 245,000 people in the United States were living with leukemia as of 2009, and more than 44,000 new cases are diagnosed each year.

The Age Factor

Chronic myeloid leukemia is the most common form of the disease among adults, and acute myeloid leukemia is the most common form among children. Although leukemia is 10 times more common in adults than children, it is the most common type of cancer in children.

Causes

Scientists do not know what causes leukemia, but it is suspected that genetic abnormalities contribute, as do environmental factors such as cigarette smoking, exposure to radiation, and/or exposure to environmental toxins or viruses.

Leukemia Symptoms

Although symptoms can vary based on where abnormal white blood cells accumulate in the body, some of the most common are swollen lymph nodes, extreme fatigue and weakness, abnormal bruising, and bleeding gums.

Diagnosis

Blood tests can determine a patient's blood cell count, and further tests such as bone marrow biopsies can confirm a diagnosis of leukemia.

Treatment

Treatment varies based on whether the leukemia is acute or chronic, the age of the patient, and the extent of the disease. Common treatments include chemotherapy, radiation, biological therapies, and bone marrow transplants.

Prognosis

Because of improved treatments, the survival rate for people with leukemia has markedly improved since the 1970s. For instance, 91 percent of children under the age of five who are diagnosed with acute lymphocytic leukemia achieve full remission.

Hope Through Research

Scientists have made remarkable progress in developing treatments that help people beat leukemia and go on to live healthy lives. As research continues, this progress will undoubtedly continue and someday may result in a cure.

Overview

"'I don't smoke. I don't drink. And I feel pretty good for 50 years old. How can I have cancer?' That's what I asked myself when doctors told me I had leukemia. I was in shock."

—Jesse Gonzalez, a leukemia survivor from Zion, Illinois.

"Leukemia cells are abnormal cells that cannot do what normal blood cells do."

—National Institutes of Health, the United States' primary agency for conducting and supporting medical research.

In August 2007 a little boy named Kaden developed a nosebleed, which was not unusual since he had been having nosebleeds for about a year. This time, however, his mother could not get the bleeding to stop, and she became concerned. Kaden's doctor ordered blood work to be done, and when the test result came back, it showed that the boy's blood was low in platelets, the cells that help blood clot in order to control bleeding. Further blood work showed that his platelet count was continuing to drop. Then Kaden developed other troubling symptoms: a fever, pain in his abdomen, and bone pain that made it difficult for him to walk. On the recommendation of a pediatric cancer specialist, Kaden underwent a bone marrow biopsy, and the diagnosis was not good—he had acute lymphocytic leukemia (ALL), a cancer of the blood and the most common type of leukemia in children. He was admitted to the hospital and several days later began chemotherapy treatments to kill the cancerous cells and hopefully return him to good health. Kaden responded very well to the treatment, and within three weeks he was in remission, meaning that his blood count had returned to normal with no sign of leukemia cells. Although he will continue to have monthly chemotherapy treatments until December 2010, he appears to be healthy, as his mother explains: "Kaden is so full of energy he is bouncing off the walls. He started preschool last week and loves it. It is so nice for him to be able to go to school and socialize with other children."[1]

What Is Leukemia?

The term *leukemia* comes from the Greek *leukos*, which means "white," and *haima*, which means "blood," and it refers to a variety of cancers that affect blood cells. In order to understand leukemia, it helps to know what blood cells are and the functions that they perform. Normal blood is made up of a fluid known as plasma, which contains three types of blood cells: red blood cells (erythrocytes), white blood cells (leukocytes), and platelets (thrombocytes). Most blood cells are produced in the soft, spongy center of bones known as bone marrow. Red blood cells carry oxygen from the lungs to tissues and organs, as well as transport carbon dioxide from the tissues back to the lungs. The function of white blood cells is to help the body fight infection and disease by killing bacteria and viruses and by working to keep the immune system healthy. Platelets are essential for proper blood clotting. If someone gets a cut on the skin, platelets collect at the site of the injury and form a plug that stops the bleeding.

> **"The term *leukemia* comes from the Greek *leukos*, which means 'white,' and *haima*, which means 'blood,' and it refers to a variety of cancers that affect blood cells."**

When cells grow old or become damaged, they naturally die (a process known as apoptosis), and new cells are formed to take their place. But in someone with leukemia, large numbers of abnormal white blood cells (known as blasts) are produced in bone marrow. The useless cells flood the bloodstream, crowding out healthy cells and preventing apoptosis from happening as it should. The American Association for Cancer Research ex-

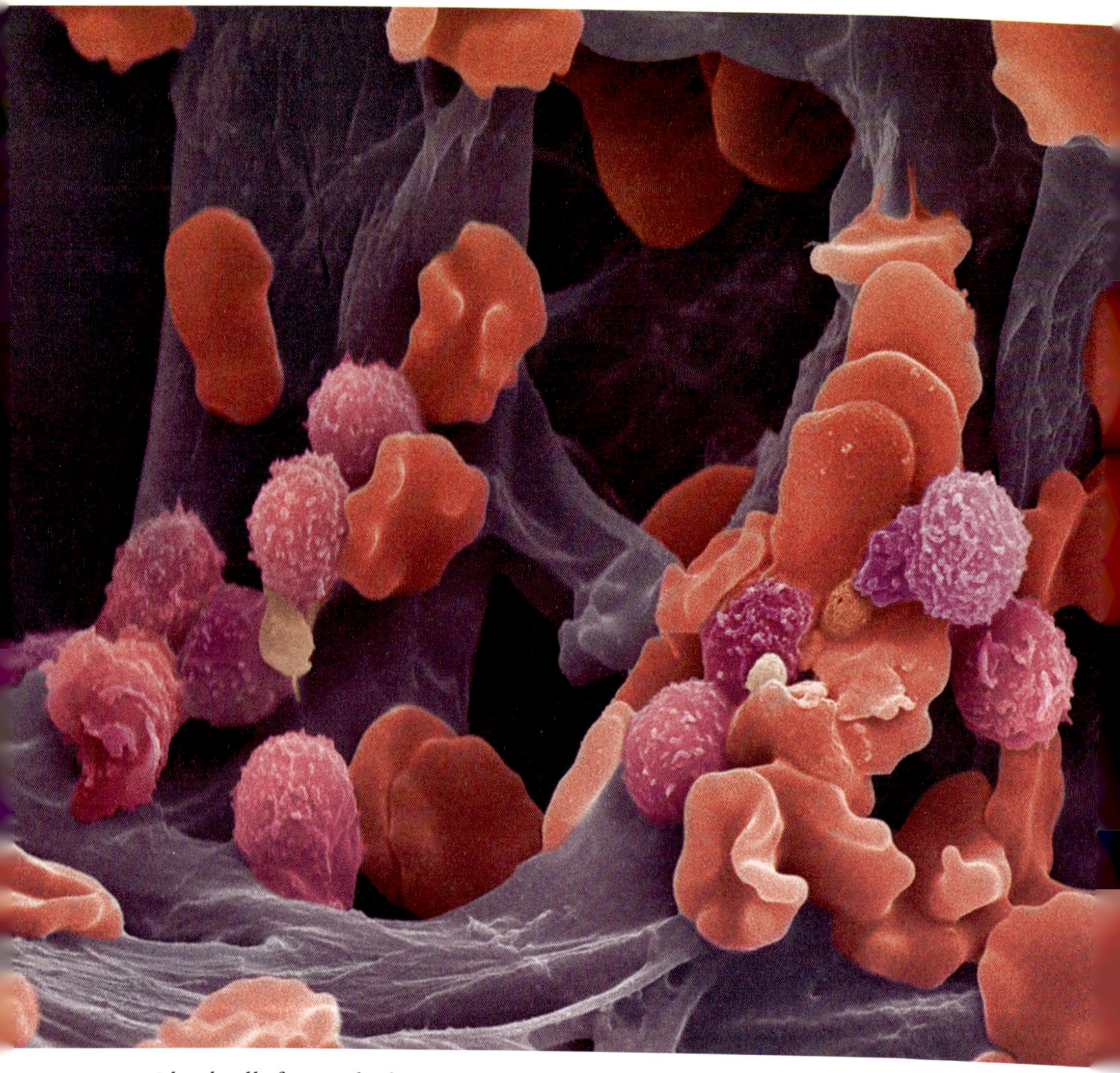

Blood cells from a leukemia patient can be seen in this colored scanning electron micrograph. This patient's leukemia is characterized by an increase in white blood cells (shown here in purple) and a decrease in red blood cells (shown here in red).

plains: "Leukemia cells overwhelm and interfere with healthy blood cells, compromising blood cell function and transporting quickly through the bloodstream."[2] When this occurs normal blood cells cannot perform their functions properly, including protecting the body against infection and bleeding.

Types of Leukemia

According to the American Society of Clinical Oncology, the various types of leukemia are named after the specific blood cell that becomes cancerous, such as the lymphocytic cells (white blood cells of the immune system) or the myeloid cells (white blood cells of the bone marrow). There are two general categories of leukemia: chronic, which develops and gets worse slowly, and acute, which develops and worsens rapidly. Within these categories, the four most common types are chronic lymphocytic leukemia (CLL), chronic myeloid (or myelogenous) leukemia (CML), acute lymphocytic (or lymphoblastic) leukemia (ALL), and acute myeloid leukemia (AML). In someone with CLL, there is an abnormal accumulation of mature lymphocytes, whereas CML is characterized by an abnormal quantity of mature myeloid cells. People who suffer from ALL have an overproduction of immature lymphocytes, while those who have AML have an abnormal quantity of immature myeloid cells.

“In addition to the common types of leukemia, there are a number of rare types, such as hairy cell leukemia.”

In addition to the common types of leukemia, there are a number of rare types, such as hairy cell leukemia. It is so named because the abnormal white blood cells have short, thin projections on their surfaces that resemble hairs when examined under a microscope. As with other forms of the disease, hairy cell leukemia results from an overproduction of abnormal white blood cells in the bloodstream. The disease is considered a chronic form of leukemia because it grows slowly and may never entirely disappear, although treatment can lead to remission.

Who Suffers from Leukemia?

The Leukemia & Lymphoma Society states that more than 245,000 people in the United States suffer from some form of leukemia. The disease strikes people of all ages, races, and nationalities, as well as both males and females. Leukemia does, however, tend to be more prevalent among males. The National Cancer Institute states that leukemia affects 15.8 per 100,000 males, and 9.5 per 100,000 females. Although leukemia is 10 times more common in adults than in children (more than half of all cases occur in people over the age of 65), it is the most common type of cancer in children. According to the Leukemia & Lymphoma Society, leukemia represents about 33 percent of all cancers in children from birth to age 14.

Hairy cell leukemia is much rarer than other types. The Mayo Clinic states that as few as 600 people in the United States are diagnosed with it each year, compared with more than 15,000 new cases of AML and over 12,000 new cases of CLL. Hairy cell leukemia affects more men than women, occurs most commonly in middle-aged or older adults, and tends not to develop in children and teenagers.

What Causes Leukemia?

Through decades of research, scientists have gained a great deal of knowledge about leukemia, including identifying the various types and learning how each affects the body. The exact causes, however, remain unknown. The National Institutes of Health (NIH) states that cancer arises from changes in chromosomes, which are long, threadlike structures that are made up of proteins and deoxyribonucleic acid (DNA), the genetic blueprint of all living things. "When the chromosomes in a cell become abnormal," the NIH writes, "the cell can lose the ability to control its growth. Sudden changes in genetic material can happen for a variety of reasons. These changes are sometimes inherited."[3]

> **"According to the Leukemia & Lymphoma Society, more than 245,000 people in the United States suffer from some form of leukemia."**

In addition to genetic factors, cellular abnormalities that lead to leukemia may occur because of environmental factors. These include cigarette smoking, exposure to high levels of radiation (such as during treatments for other forms of cancer), or exposure by industrial workers to toxins such as benzene, a clear liquid chemical that is used to make solvents, detergents, plastics, synthetic fibers, dyes, rubber, resins, paint, and many other items. Yet having one or more of these risk factors does not necessarily mean that a person will get leukemia. According to the National Cancer Institute, most people who have one or more risk factors never develop the disease.

Leukemia Symptoms

Symptoms of leukemia vary depending on where the abnormal white blood cells accumulate in the body. Some of the most common symptoms include swollen lymph nodes (especially in the neck or armpit), extreme fatigue and weakness, pain in bones or joints, and/or bleeding gums and abnormal bruising. People with acute forms of leukemia are most apt to seek medical attention early because they experience one or more of these symptoms. Those with chronic leukemia, however, often have no symptoms, and the disease may only be discovered if they undergo blood tests during a normal physical examination or suffer from unrelated health problems. This was the case with Jesse Gonzalez, who sought medical attention after he had an accidental fall at work. He explains: "I hurt my back and went to the chiropractor. He suggested I have an MRI. When the technician did the MRI, he didn't want to tell me the results. He just said, 'You need to go to the doctor right away.'"[4] Gonzalez was diagnosed with leukemia and underwent successful treatment.

> **"People who are diagnosed with acute leukemia must start treatment immediately because it can spread rapidly throughout the body."**

How Leukemia Is Diagnosed

When someone seeks medical attention for symptoms that could indicate leukemia, doctors perform a complete physical examination during which the person is checked for swelling in the lymph nodes, spleen, or liver. This is followed by blood tests that can determine the count of white blood cells, red blood cells, and platelets. If the blood test is abnormal, it may be an indication of leukemia but will not necessarily show which type of leukemia the person has. According to the NIH, to check further for leukemia cells or determine the type of leukemia, a small amount of bone and bone marrow is extracted from the patient and biopsied. If the marrow shows the presence of leukemia cells, the physician will order more tests to find out how far the disease has progressed.

Treatment of Leukemia

The recommendations for treatment vary based on whether the leukemia is chronic or acute, the age of the patient, and the extent of the disease. People who are diagnosed with acute leukemia must start treatment immediately because it can spread rapidly throughout the body. Those with chronic leukemia may opt to wait until symptoms develop (called "watchful waiting"), but in some cases that may be considered too risky, and treatment starts right away. The goal is to stop the disease from progressing so the patient is considered to be in remission. Treatment options include chemotherapy, radiation therapy, and in some cases bone marrow transplants.

During chemotherapy, one or more cancer cell–killing drugs are injected into the muscles or veins or are taken by mouth. This happens in cycles, whereby a treatment is given, a period of recovery follows, another treatment is given, and so forth. Radiation therapy (also called irradiation or radiotherapy) involves using a large machine to shoot high-energy rays that damage cancer cells and stop them from growing. If none of these treatments is successful, or the patient is at high risk for a relapse, a bone marrow transplant may be recommended. Before the procedure is performed, the patient is given high doses of chemotherapy and radiation to destroy the leukemia-producing bone marrow. Then healthy marrow (usually from a family member who is an exact match) is transplanted into the patient, and new blood cells begin to multiply in the bloodstream. The time following the transplantation is critical, and the patient usually stays in the hospital for several weeks until it is confirmed that healthy white blood cells are being produced. Otherwise, he or she is susceptible to serious infection.

Side Effects of Leukemia Treatment

Aggressive leukemia therapies often damage healthy cells and tissue, so undergoing treatment can be extremely hard on someone who suffers from the disease. Common side effects of chemotherapy and radiation include infections, hair loss (both body hair and scalp hair), nausea and vomiting, and sores in the mouth. Because chemotherapy decreases the

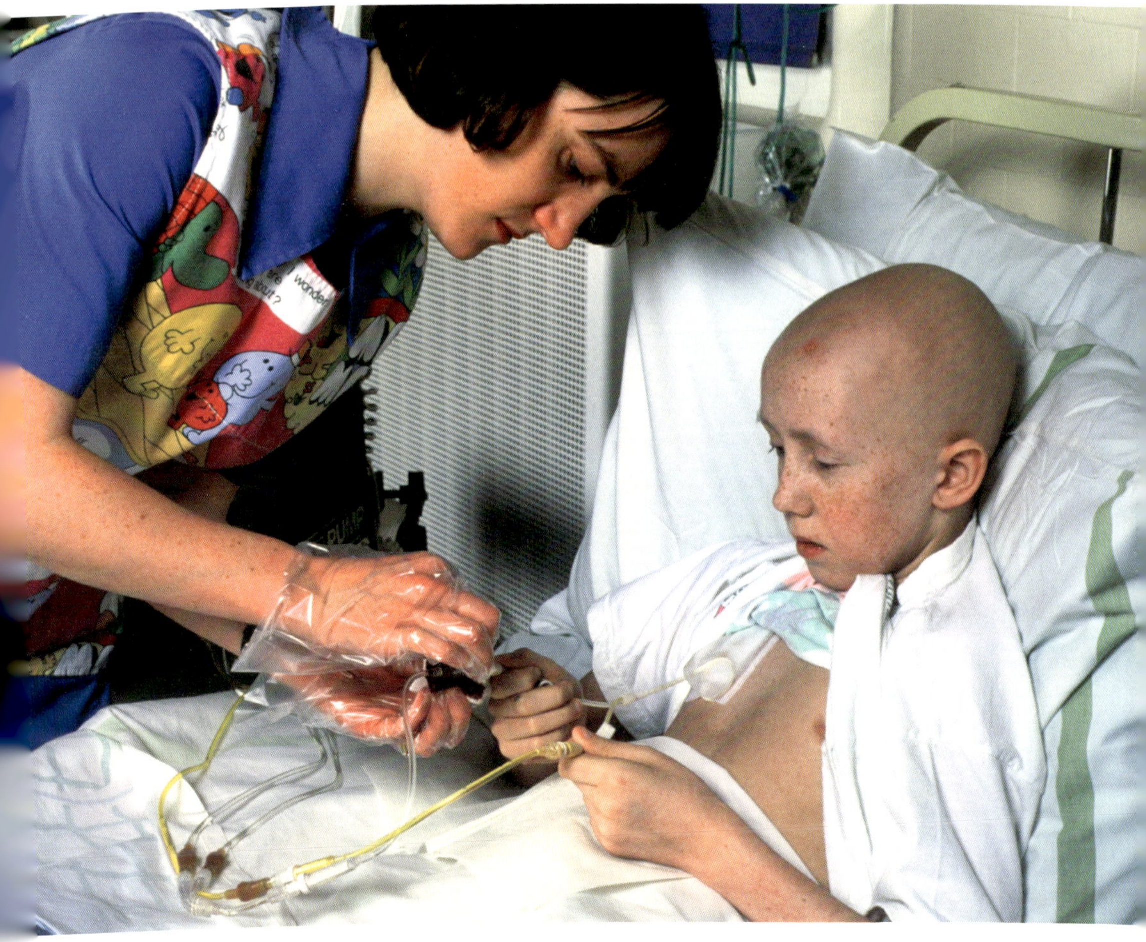

A nurse adjusts an intravenous line that delivers chemotherapy drugs to a boy who is being treated for leukemia. Leukemia is the most common form of cancer in children.

number of platelets in the blood, this can result in nosebleeds, bleeding gums, or passing blood in the urine or stool. Young children who have leukemia cells in the brain and undergo radiation therapy to kill the cells may develop learning disabilities and problems with coordination.

Side effects from leukemia treatments are not limited to physical problems—many people also suffer psychologically because of fear and stress. According to Debra Ochs, who was diagnosed with AML in 2003, the psychological stress was worse than the physical effects of chemotherapy. She explains: "From the time you wake up in the morning

> **Aggressive leukemia therapies often damage healthy cells and tissue, so undergoing treatment can be extremely hard on someone who suffers from the disease.**

to the time you go to bed at night, it is always there. Even when you are sleeping, you dream about what's going on. You constantly wonder: Is that the same feeling I had in my back before? Is that the same twinge? You worry about what will happen if you don't make it, especially what will happen to your family."[5]

A number of side effects can also result from bone marrow transplants, such as life-threatening infections. By far the most dangerous risk of bone marrow transplants is graft-versus-host disease (GvHD), in which the transplanted cells attack the patient's healthy tissue. This happened to a young boy named Elijah Poolman, who underwent a bone marrow transplant in October 2002 because he was considered a high risk for a leukemia relapse. After the surgery he developed GvHD when immune cells in the transplanted marrow from the donor (his older brother Isaac) attacked Elijah's vital organs. Doctors at the Mayo Clinic were able to treat the condition, and Elijah made a complete recovery. This is not always the case, however, as the most severe cases of GvHD can be fatal.

How Successful Are Leukemia Treatments?

In the past, people who were diagnosed with leukemia almost certainly faced death, but medical science has resulted in treatments that successfully fight the disease. According to the Leukemia & Lymphoma Society, in the early 1960s a patient with leukemia only had a 14 percent chance of living 5 years. Today, after treatment, the average survival rate is 51 percent and is much higher for some leukemia types. For instance, the survival rate for CLL is 76 percent, and for children who are diagnosed with ALL under the age of 5, it is 91 percent.

Yet even though many people show no signs of leukemia after treatment, it is not the same as a cure because cancerous cells can return later. If that happens leukemia may again flare up, and the patient will suffer a relapse. That is what happened to Georgina Horlock, a little girl from the United

Kingdom who was diagnosed with leukemia at the age of two. After nine weeks of intensive treatment, Georgina's health had markedly improved, and she was able to go to nursery school. Her mother took samples of her blood each week and dropped it off at the laboratory for testing, and the results indicated a normal white blood cell count. Then when Georgina was 12 years old, she had a relapse and underwent a bone marrow transplant. After contracting a serious infection, her health rapidly deteriorated and she died. "Basically, she had been too heavily treated by that stage," her mother writes. "Her body just began to fall apart. It was desperate and terrible."[6]

What Are the Prospects for Preventing or Curing Leukemia?

Leukemia research is being aggressively pursued by scientists so they can learn more about how cancerous cells develop and when they start to develop. The hope is that this research will someday prevent the disease or lead to a cure, rather than just produce treatments that lead to remission. According to the American Association for Cancer Research (AACR), the development of combinations of drugs that target particular proteins in leukemia cells is a major area of research and discovery. "As researchers continue to better understand the molecular events leading to leukemia," the AACR states, "they continue to work towards specific drugs that will halt the disease's progression. . . . Researchers also continue to work to improve other leukemia treatments."[7] In June 2007, scientists announced that a drug already proven safe in humans may be able to help increase the number of stem cells, which are the master cells of the body from which all other cells are produced. This treatment may help to improve the effectiveness of stem cell transplants.

> **"By far the most dangerous risk of bone marrow transplants is graft-versus-host disease (GvHD), in which the transplanted cells attack the patient's healthy tissue."**

In 2008 scientists from the United Kingdom announced a research breakthrough that led to a new understanding of the causes of childhood leukemia. The study involved four-year-old identical twins, Olivia and Isabella Murphy. An analysis of the girls' blood showed that both had genetic mutations in stem cells found in bone marrow. Because neither of their parents had the same mutation, it likely occurred while they were still in the womb. Only Olivia developed leukemia, however, because she suffered a second mutation sometime after she was born, which was possibly caused by an infection.

By studying the differences in the twins' blood, scientists were able to pinpoint the pre-leukemic cells in both of them, and then figure out the sequence of the genetic mutations. This discovery will enable the doctors to monitor Isabella (and other children like her) closely to determine whether her pre-leukemic stem cells develop the additional mutation. If that happens, her leukemia will be caught early enough for treatment to be started and the cancerous cells to be destroyed before they spread throughout her body. "The crucial question is in which cells does this start," says scientist Tariq Enver. "What is the critical hit? Isabella gave us an opportunity almost to look back in time, to see which cells the cancer begins in."[8] Enver adds that the research team's next goal is to target both the pre-leukemic cells and the cancerous cells with new or existing drugs to cure the leukemia, while avoiding the harsh, often debilitating effects of chemotherapy and other cancer treatments.

Decades of Progress

From the early 1960s, when a diagnosis of leukemia was viewed as a death sentence, to the present time, when the chance of survival has improved dramatically, much progress has been made in the fight against leukemia. Researcher Emil J. Freireich explains: "Just 50 years ago, the diagnosis of acute leukemia was a death warrant. Patients looked forward to an immediate onset of bleeding from mouth, nose, urine, rectum, major infection, and a lifespan of approximately two months on average, with virtually 100% mortality by one year after diagnosis."[9] Today children who develop leukemia at a young age have an excellent chance of going into full remission, and the prognosis has also markedly improved for adults. There is still a long way to go, however, because many people die from leukemia. With continued research, the odds of surviving the disease may improve, and there may come a time when it can be prevented and/or cured. For those who suffer from leukemia, that would be the best news they could ever hope to hear.

What Is Leukemia?

"Leukemia is often referred to as cancer of the blood. It is characterized by the widespread uncontrolled proliferation of large numbers of abnormal blood cells, usually white blood cells, which take over the bone marrow and quickly spread to the blood stream."

—Leukemia Research Foundation, which funds research into the causes and cures of leukemia and related disorders.

"Leukemia forms in several different types of white blood cells (lymphocytes, granulocytes and monocytes), which are responsible for fighting infection."

—American Association for Cancer Research, whose mission is to prevent and cure cancer through research, education, communication, and collaboration.

On October 1, 1845, the *Edinburgh Medical and Surgical Journal* published a paper that was written by John Hughes Bennett, an English physician and pathologist. In the paper Bennett described two of his patients who died after their spleens became enlarged, and he said their deaths were caused by "purulent matter" (pus) in their bloodstreams. He named the mysterious disease leucocythaemia, and more than a century later was credited by the Leukemia Research Fund for being the first person to describe leukemia. But a year before Bennett's work was published, a French physician named Alfred Donné had provided a more accurate description of the disease in his book entitled *Complimentary Course on Microscopy for Medical Studies*. In a chapter called "Alterations of the White Blood Cells," Donné acknowledged that white blood cells resembled purulent matter, but upon closer examination were not pus at all. "Several cases exist with a great excess of white blood cells," he wrote. "Blood of such patients contains so many white blood cells that at first glance I thought they contained purulent matter. In fact, I believe that the excess of white blood cells is due to an arrest of maturation of blood."[10]

"The three main types of blood cancer are lymphoma, myeloma, and leukemia, which together account for nearly 900,000 cases in the United States."

Donné had previously corresponded with a colleague regarding blood samples of another patient who died with an enlarged spleen, which indicated the presence of excessive white blood cells. Then, too, he correctly determined that the patient had died of an unknown disease that was caused by abnormally large amounts of immature (and therefore useless) white blood cells. Throughout the following years, Donné repeatedly denounced the erroneous theory that leukemia was caused by purulent matter in the blood. But according to author and physician Laurent Degos, in spite of Donné's many accomplishments, including being the first to discover the connection between white blood cells and leukemia, he was never formally recognized by his peers.

When Blood Turns Cancerous

According to the American Cancer Society, hundreds of varieties of cancer exist, but only certain types affect the production and function of blood cells. The three main types of blood cancer are lymphoma, myeloma, and leukemia, which together account for nearly 900,000 cases in the United States. Leukemia is the second most common form of blood cancer (after lymphoma) and strikes more than 40,000 adults and children every year. Although many people who are treated survive leukemia and go on to live healthy lives, the Leukemia & Lymphoma Society states that the disease remains the sixth most common cause of cancer deaths in men and the seventh in women.

Leukemia occurs because large numbers of abnormal white blood cells are produced in bone marrow. These cells do not have the same appearance as normal white blood cells, nor do they function the way they should. Instead, the abnormal cells multiply and crowd out healthy white blood cells, red blood cells, and platelets. As a result, white blood cells lose their ability to fight infection and disease, red blood cells cannot properly transport oxygen throughout the body, and platelets lose their ability to cause blood to clot.

Jonathan O'Malley is a young leukemia patient from Lumberton, Texas. In August 2008 he was treated at a hospital emergency room for a sore throat, and doctors diagnosed tonsillitis. A blood test by a specialist, however, showed that Jonathan had a much more serious disease—leukemia. His mother, Melanie O'Malley, was sitting at a stoplight when her cell phone rang and she received the frightening news. "I will never forget that red light," she says. "The doctor called and said that normal blood count of white blood cells is between 5,000 and 13,000. Jonathan's was 230,000. His blood was 96 percent leukemia."[11] Jonathan underwent 9 months of intensive treatments, including chemotherapy, and spent over 240 days in the hospital. As of June 2009, at the age of 17, his leukemia was in complete remission, although it will be 5 years before he is officially declared cancer free.

Acute Forms of Leukemia

According to the Princeton University database of English, the word *acute* is defined as "having or experiencing a rapid onset and short but severe course" or "extremely sharp or intense."[12] In describing acute leukemias, such descriptions are apt because symptoms develop and worsen quickly, in a period of time as short as several weeks or even days. Acute leukemias involve the production of abnormal white blood cells that develop and multiply rapidly and can flood the bloodstream, rendering someone with acute leukemia gravely ill in a short period of time. The American Association for Cancer Research states that in acute types of leukemia, genetic mutations in stem cells result in an excess of immature, useless white blood cells in bone marrow and blood. As the abnormal blood cells continue to crowd out the production of healthy cells, normal cell function is disrupted and the leukemia grows worse at a fast rate of speed. One main type of acute leukemia, acute myeloid leukemia (AML), is most prevalent among people who are 55 and older. The Leukemia & Lymphoma Society states that AML incidence increases dramatically among the elderly and is most prevalent among those who are in their seventies and above. But even though it is uncommon, the disease strikes younger people as well. Jonathan O'Malley suffered from AML, and doctors told his parents that on average, only about 500 cases develop in children and adolescents each year.

> **Acute leukemias involve the production of abnormal white blood cells that develop and multiply rapidly and can flood the bloodstream, rendering someone with acute leukemia gravely ill in a short period of time.**

As with AML, acute lymphocytic leukemia (ALL) can affect people of all ages, but this form of leukemia is most prevalent among children under the age of 10 and adults older than 50. According to the American Cancer Society, only about 1 percent of new cancer diagnoses affect children. But among children and youth who *do* develop cancer, more than one-third suffer from leukemia, and an estimated 70 percent of those have ALL. In June 2006, 2-year-old Lauren Richmond was diagnosed with ALL, and in 2007 her 4-year-old sister was diagnosed with the same disease, which is extremely unusual among siblings who are not identical twins. "It was quite a shock,"[13] says the girls' mother, referring to her reaction at hearing the diagnosis. Yet in spite of all that the girls have endured because of their disease and the harsh side effects of treatment, doctors are optimistic that they will both make a full recovery.

Chronic Leukemias

As indicated by the word *chronic*, which means "long lasting," chronic forms of leukemia progress much more slowly than acute leukemias. That is because in someone with chronic lymphocytic leukemia (CLL) or chronic myeloid leukemia (CML), the excess white blood cells created in bone marrow are mature and initially function in much the same way as healthy white blood cells. Over a period of time, though, this changes. The Leukemia & Lymphoma Society states that CLL starts with a change to a single lymphocyte. The abnormal cells multiply until they begin to replace healthy lymphocytes in bone marrow and lymph nodes and eventually overcrowd the bloodstream, causing normal cells to lose their ability to fight infection. Although CLL can strike people of any age, the majority of people who develop it are 50 years of age or older. It is the most common form of adult leukemia in the United States and other western countries.

“Some kinds of leukemia occur much more rarely than others. One example is juvenile myelomonocytic leukemia (JMML), which most commonly strikes children under the age of 4.”

CML is also a slow-growing form of leukemia, but it develops differently from CLL. People with CML have what is known as the Philadelphia chromosome, which forms when pieces of chromosome 22 and chromosome 9 break off and switch places. This abnormality results in the formation of a cancer gene called BCR-ABL. Once the cancer gene has formed, it gives instructions to the cell in which it is contained to begin making tyrosine kinase, a protein that leads to an overproduction of abnormal white blood cells. When these abnormal cells flood the bloodstream, the result is the development of CML. Like CLL, most people who develop CML are over the age of 50. But even though it is extremely rare in those who are younger, people of any age can develop it. Jason Blake was diagnosed with CML in October 2007 when he was 34 years old. A professional hockey player from Toronto, Canada, Blake choked back tears when he made the announcement to his fellow teammates, but he was assured by his doctors that his form of leukemia was highly treatable. He began taking daily medication that has been shown to be effective in treating CML. As of 2009, Blake's prognosis was excellent, and he remained a top goal scorer for his team, the Toronto Maple Leafs.

Rare Leukemia Types

Some kinds of leukemia occur much more rarely than others. One example is juvenile myelomonocytic leukemia (JMML), which most commonly strikes children under the age of 4. According to the Juvenile Myelomonocytic Leukemia Foundation, JMML only accounts for about 1 to 2 percent of childhood leukemias each year. It begins in myeloid blood cells and falls somewhere between chronic and acute—it does not grow as fast as AML, nor does it grow as slowly as CML. Scientists have determined that about 80 percent of JMML patients have some sort of genetic abnormality that has been linked to development of this rare form of leukemia.

> **"Although a diagnosis of any form of leukemia meant certain death in the past, many people now survive much longer than was ever believed to be possible."**

Adolfo Gonzalez Jr. was only 13 months old when he was diagnosed with JMML, and doctors told the boy's parents that with or without treatment, he would not survive. Leukemia specialist Gary Kleiner explains: "Most of the cases are fatal by the time the child is three years old."[14] Adolfo beat the odds, however. After undergoing chemotherapy and an experimental stem cell transplant using a donor's umbilical cord blood, the little boy was still cancer free as of January 2009.

Michael Staub was also stricken with a rare form of leukemia—but he was not as fortunate as Adolfo. When he was 20, Staub was diagnosed with a rare hybrid form of ALL and AML, a combination that markedly increased his resistance to chemotherapy. After undergoing the first 2 rounds, he took a turn for the worse in August 2001 and was readmitted to the hospital for a third round. Afterward Staub returned home with his parents while the 3 of them awaited the test results. A few weeks later they got the bad news: The chemotherapy had not worked. His mother asked the cancer specialist when Staub would undergo the next round and was shocked to hear his answer: "There's no next round," the doctor said. "Michael's incurable. He's dying."[15] On April 15, 2002, Michael Staub lost his battle with leukemia and died peacefully at his home.

The Dreaded "C" Word

Of the hundreds of types of cancers that exist, leukemia is among those that affect blood cells. All forms of the disease result from overproduction of useless white blood cells, but in people with acute leukemias, the abnormal cells develop and multiply much more rapidly than in those with chronic types. Although a diagnosis of any form of leukemia meant certain death in the past, many people now survive much longer than was ever believed to be possible. Yet even with all the progress that has been made in leukemia research, and with life expectancies for people who suffer from the disease dramatically higher than in recent decades, for someone to hear "you have cancer" is still shocking as well as frightening.

For those who are living with leukemia or have family members who suffer from it, there is no choice but to hope for the best and try not to dwell on fear and dread. That is the philosophy of Katie Caskey, whose two-year-old son, Carson, has leukemia. She and her husband say they have learned to take life one day at a time, as she explains: "Each week that he doesn't relapse, that just gives you hope. . . . I don't know that I will ever be at peace with my son having leukemia. It's our life, so I live it. I used to cry every day. Now, I don't."[16]

Primary Source Quotes*

What Is Leukemia?

"Leukemia is cancer of blood-forming tissue such as the bone marrow. Types of leukemia are grouped by the type of cell affected and by the rate of cell growth."

—M.D. Anderson Cancer Center, "Living with Leukemia," August 20, 2008. www.mdanderson.org.

The M.D. Anderson Cancer Center, which is headquartered in Houston, Texas, seeks to eliminate cancer through programs that integrate patient care, research, prevention, and education.

"Anyone can get leukemia. Leukemia affects all ages and sexes."

—Leukemia & Lymphoma Society, "Leukemia Facts & Statistics," June 17, 2009. www.leukemia-lymphoma.org.

Through blood research, education, and patient services, the Leukemia & Lymphoma Society seeks to cure leukemia, lymphoma, Hodgkin's disease, and myeloma and to improve the quality of life of patients and their families.

* Editor's Note: While the definition of a primary source can be narrowly or broadly defined, for the purposes of Compact Research, a primary source consists of: 1) results of original research presented by an organization or researcher; 2) eyewitness accounts of events, personal experience, or work experience; 3) first-person editorials offering pundits' opinions; 4) government officials presenting political plans and/or policies; 5) representatives of organizations presenting testimony or policy.

“When a child has leukemia, large numbers of abnormal white blood cells are produced in the bone marrow. These abnormal white cells crowd the bone marrow and flood the bloodstream, but they cannot perform their proper role of protecting the body against disease because they are defective.”

—Robin E. Miller, “Childhood Cancer: Leukemia,” KidsHealth, June 2007. http://kidshealth.org.

Miller is a pediatrician in the division of hematology/oncology at Alfred I. duPont Hospital for Children in Wilmington, Delaware.

“Leukemia isn’t just a children’s disease. It has four main types and many subtypes—and only some are common among children.”

—Mayo Clinic, “Leukemia,” April 5, 2008. www.mayoclinic.com.

The Mayo Clinic is a world-renowned medical practice that is dedicated to the diagnosis and treatment of virtually every type of complex illness.

“Acute myelocytic leukemia (AML) is the most common type of leukemia among adults, although it affects people of all ages.”

—Emil J. Freireich, “Acute Myelocytic Leukemia (AML),” Merck Manuals, June 2008. www.merck.com.

Freireich is a professor of medicine and director of the adult leukemia research program at M.D. Anderson Cancer Center in Houston, Texas.

“Unlike normal blood cells, leukemia cells don’t die when they should. They may crowd out normal white blood cells, red blood cells, and platelets. This makes it hard for normal blood cells to do their work.”

—National Cancer Institute, “What You Need to Know About Leukemia,” September 2008. www.cancer.gov.

The National Cancer Institute, which is an agency of the National Institutes of Health, is the U.S. government’s principal federal agency for cancer research and training.

“Leukemia is different from other types of cancer that start in organs such as the lungs, colon, or breast and then spread to the bone marrow. Cancers that start elsewhere and then spread to the bone marrow are not leukemia.”

—American Cancer Society, “What Is Chronic Lymphocytic Leukemia?” May 14, 2009. www.cancer.org.

The American Cancer Society seeks to eliminate cancer as a major health problem by preventing it and saving lives through research, education, advocacy, and service.

“Chronic myeloid leukemia (CML) is a cancer of blood cells, characterized by replacement of the bone marrow with malignant, leukemic cells.”

—National Institutes of Health, “Blood and Lymph Diseases,” January 14, 2009. www.ncbi.nlm.nih.gov.

The National Institutes of Health is the United States’ primary agency for conducting and supporting medical research.

“Leukemia strikes males and females of all ages and all races. It does not discriminate.”

—Leukemia Research Foundation, “About Us: Microscope,” 2008. www.leukemia-research.org.

The mission of the Leukemia Research Foundation is to conquer leukemia and other blood cancers by funding research into their causes and cures.

What Is Leukemia?

- According to the Leukemia & Lymphoma Society, leukemia is one of **the top 15 most frequently occurring cancers** in all races or ethnicities.
- The National Institutes of Health states that leukemia occurs because cancerous cells that form in bone marrow **crowd out healthy cells**, which disrupts their ability to fight off infection and function normally.
- A 2009 report by the Leukemia & Lymphoma Society states that an estimated **245,225 people** in the United States are living with, or are in remission from, leukemia.
- The most common type of leukemia in adults is chronic lymphocytic leukemia, with an estimated **15,110 cases** diagnosed during 2009.
- The most common type of leukemia in young children is **acute lymphocytic leukemia** (ALL); the Leukemia & Lymphoma Society states that the incidence of ALL among 1- to 4-year-olds is more than 9 times greater than the rate for young adults aged 20 to 24.
- The Leukemia Research Foundation states that **121 Americans are diagnosed with leukemia every day**, and **every 10 minutes someone dies from leukemia** or another form of blood cancer.
- Chronic leukemias, which generally strike older adults, account for **11 percent** more cases than acute leukemias.

Leukemia in the United States

According to the American Cancer Society, there are hundreds of types of cancer and leukemia is among those that affect the blood. As this graph illustrates, there are a number of cancers that are far more prevalent, but nearly 45,000 people are diagnosed with leukemia in the United States every year.

Estimated new cancer cases in the United States—2009

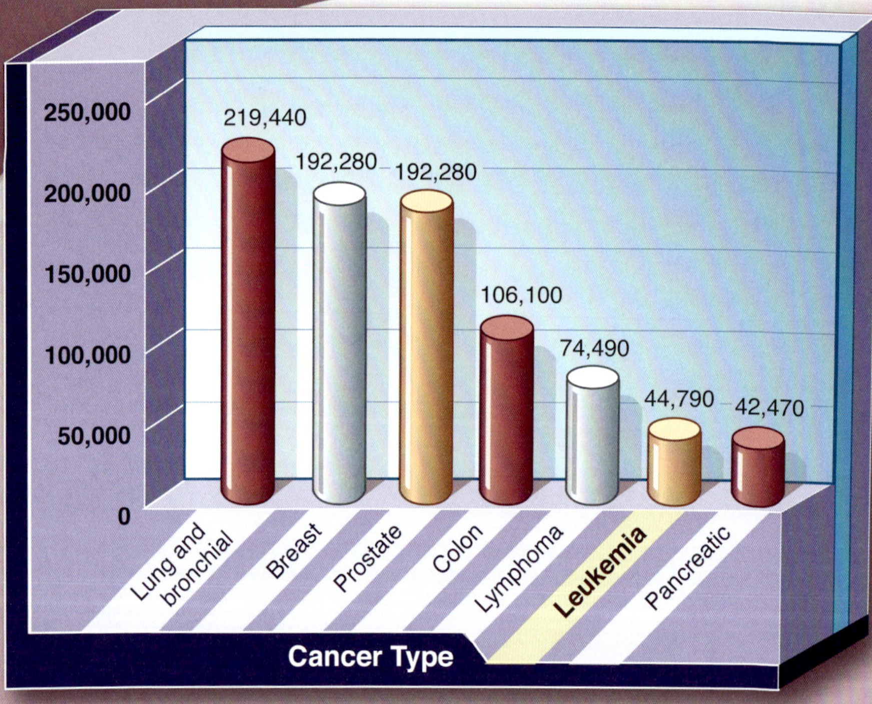

Source: American Cancer Society, "Cancer Facts & Figures 2009," 2009. www.cancer.org.

- The median patient age at diagnosis of chronic leukemias is **67 years**.
- Studies have shown that leukemia accounts for about **33 percent** of cancer cases in children from birth to age 14.

Leukemia More Prevalent Among Males than Females

Leukemia can strike anyone, anywhere, regardless of age, race, or nationality. Although scientists cannot explain why, every type of leukemia is more common among males than females.

Estimated number of new leukemia cases in the United States during 2008

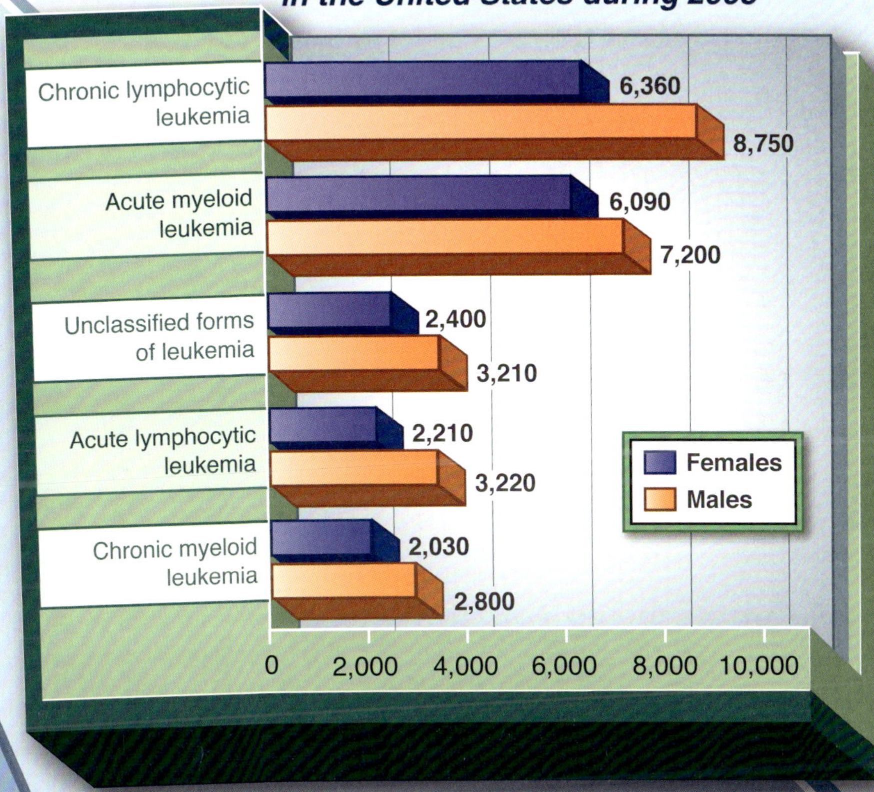

Source: Leukemia & Lymphoma Society, "Facts 2008–2009," June 2008. www.leukemia-lymphoma.org.

- The American Cancer Society states that at least **20 percent** of people with chronic leukemia have no symptoms at the time their cancer is diagnosed.

Leukemia Is the Most Common Childhood Cancer

Many types of cancer are far more prevalent than leukemia among the general population. But leukemia is the most common of all cancers from birth to age 19.

Most common types of cancer among children and youth from birth to age 19*

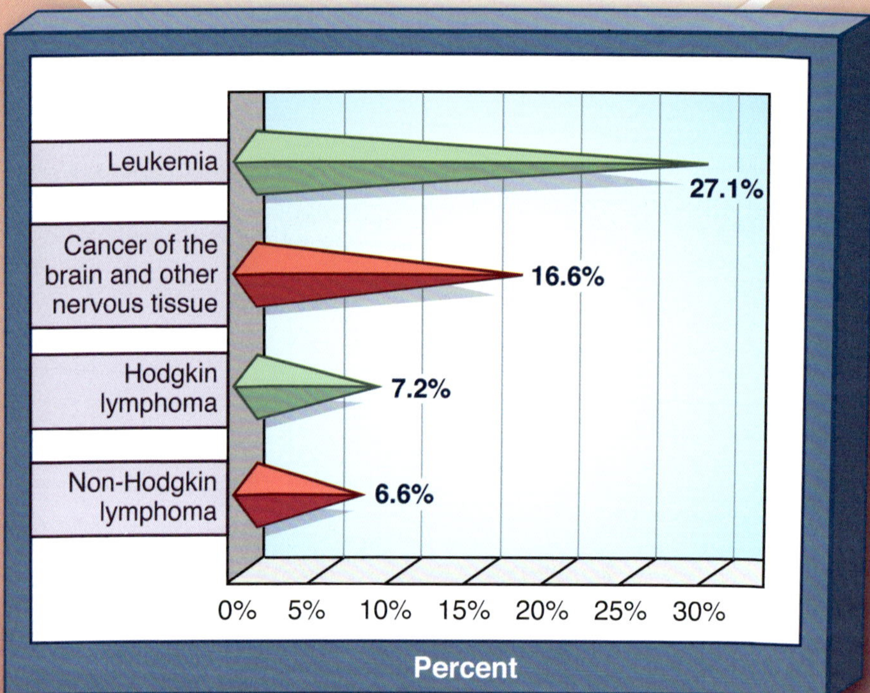

*Expressed as a percent of all childhood cancers

Source: Leukemia & Lymphoma Society, "Leukemia Facts & Statistics," July 1, 2009. www.leukemia-lymphoma.org.

- According to the Leukemia & Lymphoma Society, leukemia incidence is **highest among Caucasians** and lowest among American Indians, Alaskan natives, and Asian and Pacific Islander populations.

The Creation and Functions of Blood Cells

The human body contains trillions of cells that work together to perform crucial functions such as helping blood to clot and fighting infection and disease. In someone with leukemia, the bloodstream is flooded with abnormal cells that inhibit the normal blood cells' ability to do their work properly. This illustration shows how blood cells form and their functions within the body.

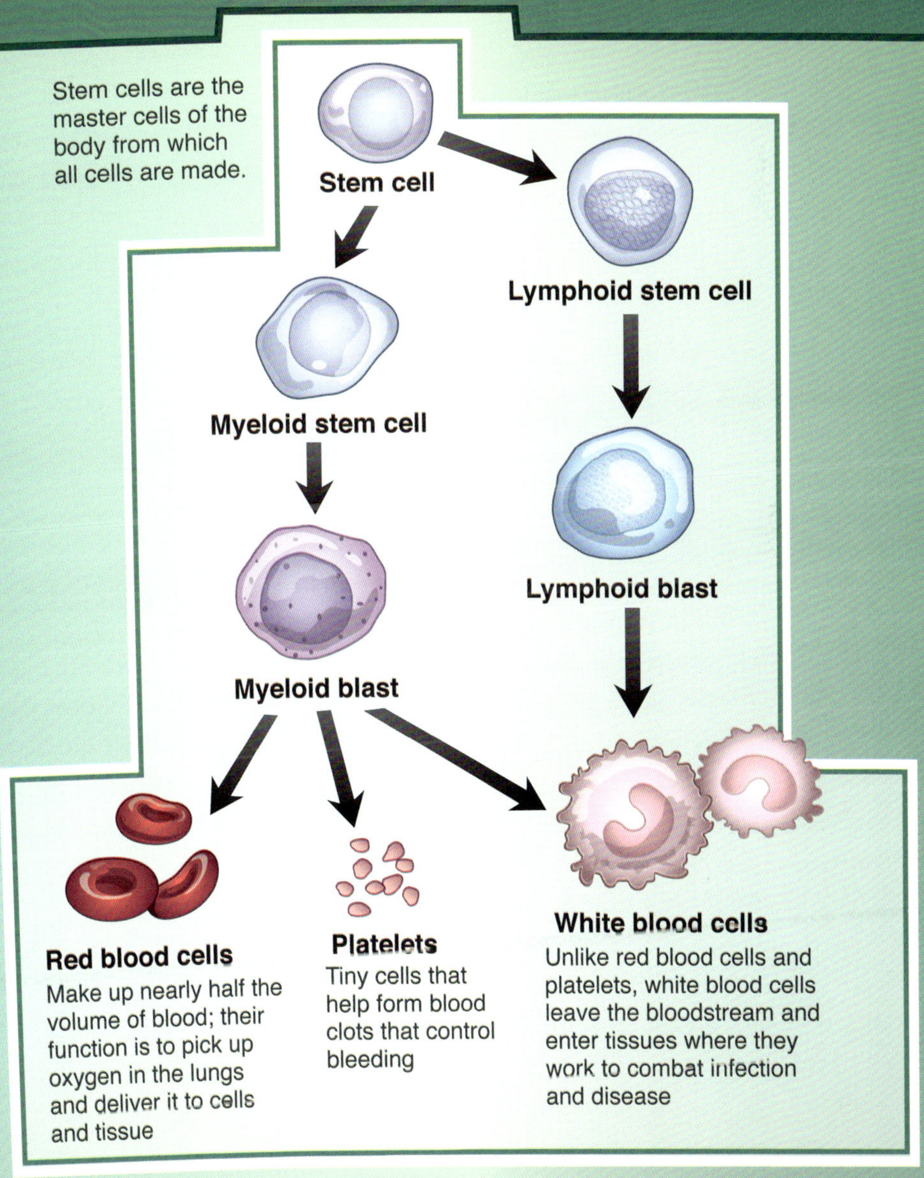

Sources: National Cancer Institute, "What You Need to Know About Leukemia," September 2008. www.cancer.gov; Leukemia & Lymphoma Society, "Blood Marrow Stem Cell Transplantation," February 2008. www.leukemia-lymphoma.org.

What Causes Leukemia?

"The specific cause of leukemia is still not known. Scientists suspect that viral, genetic, environmental or immunologic factors may be involved."

—M.D. Anderson Cancer Center, which seeks to eliminate cancer through programs that integrate patient care, research, prevention, and education.

"Most people with known risk factors don't get leukemia. And many people with leukemia have none of these risk factors."

—Mayo Clinic, a world-renowned medical practice that is dedicated to the diagnosis and treatment of virtually every type of complex illness.

Even with all that is known about cancer, it is still mysterious for many reasons, and leukemia is certainly no exception. Scientists wonder, even with a variety of risk factors, why do so many people not develop leukemia while others *are* stricken with it? The American Cancer Society states that although some people with leukemia have one or more known risk factors, the majority do not, meaning that the cause of their disease cannot be identified. The society explains: "Even when a patient has one or more risk factors, there is no way to tell whether it actually caused the cancer. And, many people with one or more cancer risk factors never develop this disease."[17]

The American Cancer Society adds that in recent years, scientists have made a great deal of progress in understanding how certain changes in DNA can potentially cause normal bone marrow cells to become leukemic cells. For instance, some genes contain instructions for controlling cell growth and division, while the function of others is to slow down cell division or cause cells to die at the appropriate time. It is possible that mutations in these genes can lead to leukemia and/or other types of cancer, but how and why the abnormalities occur is largely a mystery.

Is Leukemia Hereditary?

Scientists have long known that certain cancers, such as those of the breast, ovaries, colon, and prostate, tend to run in families. Although this is also true of leukemia, hereditary forms of the disease are rare. According to the American Cancer Society, genetic mutations play a role in whether someone develops leukemia, but most cases of leukemia are not caused by inherited mutations: "Usually," the organization writes, "DNA mutations related to leukemia develop after conception rather than having been inherited. Some of these acquired mutations may occur early, even before birth."[18]

Hereditary genetic mutations, however, have been linked to some cases of leukemia. In 2007 researchers from Ohio State University's Comprehensive Cancer Center announced that they had discovered the first inherited mutated gene that increases someone's risk for developing chronic lymphocytic leukemia (CLL). The mutation was found in DAPK1, a gene that normally helps trigger the death of cells through the natural process of apoptosis. After analyzing the DNA of a family in which the father, four sons, a grandson, and a distant female relative developed CLL, the scientists identified the mutated gene in all of them. They determined that the mutation significantly reduced the gene's ability to function properly, and they also found that a chemical change (not hereditary) took place that effectively switched the gene off and rendered it useless in controlling cell growth. When this happens, it leads to the production of abnormal cells in bone marrow and blood and the onset of leukemia.

Genetic Disorders and Leukemia

Even though hereditary forms of leukemia are rare, people who are born with certain genetic disorders have an elevated risk of developing the disease. One example is Down syndrome. For reasons that are not fully understood, children who are born with the disorder are at higher risk of developing leukemia than children who do not have it. According to the

National Down Syndrome Society, 1 in every 100 children with Down syndrome develops leukemia, compared with 1 in every 2,000 children who get the disease and do not have Down syndrome. This was the case with a little girl named Chantel, who was born with Down syndrome and developed leukemia when she was 17 months old. After 9 months of chemotherapy, Chantel was declared to be in remission in 1999—and as of January 2009, she had been a leukemia survivor for 10 years. This is typical of many children with Down syndrome. Scientists say that they have substantially higher survival rates, as well as lower relapse rates, than children without the disorder. Some studies have suggested an ironic reason for this: The same chromosomal abnormalities that cause Down syndrome may somehow strengthen the immune systems of those who have it, so they respond better to leukemia treatments.

> **According to the American Cancer Society, genetic mutations play a role in whether someone develops leukemia, but most cases of leukemia are not caused by inherited mutations.**

Much rarer than Down syndrome is a genetic disorder known as Bloom's syndrome, which results from a hereditary gene mutation. Since the disorder was identified in 1954, fewer than 300 people have been diagnosed with it worldwide, and it is most common among Jews of eastern European descent. "Bloomies," as those who have Bloom's syndrome often call themselves, have chromosomal abnormalities that lead to stunted growth, hypersensitivity to sunlight that causes painful sores on the skin, sterility, and immune system deficiencies that leave them susceptible to many forms of cancer, especially leukemia and lymphoma. Sheryl Grossman was diagnosed with Bloom's syndrome when she was 1 year old. Now at age 32, she is just 49 inches tall (124cm) and weighs only 46 pounds (21kg). "I hate walking down the street, especially on St. Patrick's Day," she says. "People pat me on the head and ask for wishes, like I'm a leprechaun. It's hard to go to public places where there are exhibits. I become one. People are there to look at things that are unusual, only I'm not in a cage or behind glass."[19]

Most people with Bloom's syndrome develop leukemia or other cancers by the time they are in their mid twenties, and they die young—usually by the age of 48.

The Role of Environment

Although most people who have genetic mutations that predispose them to developing leukemia never get the disease, certain environmental factors increase their risk. For example, exposure to high levels of radiation has been closely linked with childhood leukemia. According to the American Cancer Society, survivors of the atomic bomb explosions in Japan in 1945 "had a 20-fold increased risk of developing AML, usually within 6 to 8 years after exposure."[20] People can also be exposed to radiation in other ways, such as when radiation therapy is used to treat other forms of cancer. The American Cancer Society states that children and adults who undergo radiation therapy and/or chemotherapy have a higher risk of developing leukemia later in life, usually within 5 to 10 years of treatment.

Along with radiation, another environmental factor that has been linked to leukemia is exposure to toxic chemicals such as benzene, a colorless, flammable liquid with a sweet odor. In the United States benzene is widely used in industrial operations, most often as a solvent and as a starting material for the production of other chemicals. According to the American Cancer Society, the greatest risk of exposure to high levels of benzene is to people who work in the rubber industry, oil refineries, chemical plants, shoe manufacturing, and gasoline-related industrial operations. Studies of workers in these industries have shown a link between exposure to benzene and leukemia, most commonly AML and CLL. After developing AML in 2006, a woman from Illinois filed a lawsuit against her former employers, claiming that her leukemia was caused by exposure to benzene-containing

"Most people with Bloom's syndrome develop leukemia or other cancers by the time they are in their mid twenties, and they die young—usually by the age of 48."

products in the workplace. Although she acknowledged that the areas where she worked were labeled "Benzene-Regulated Areas," she said she was not made aware of the dangers of the chemical, nor was she provided with adequate protection.

A similar lawsuit was filed by a Texas man in 2009. After working for more than 30 years at an Amoco refinery, during which time he was exposed to benzene in solvents and chemicals, he was diagnosed with CLL in May 2006. He, too, claimed that he was not aware of the dangers associated with benzene, nor was he given any protection from his employer to reduce his exposure to it.

The Virus Connection

Some studies have shown that exposure to certain viruses elevates the risk of developing leukemia. For instance, T-cell leukemia virus type 1, which is a distant cousin of the human immunovirus (HIV) that leads to AIDS, is linked to a very rare form of leukemia known as adult T-cell lymphocytic leukemia. According to the National Cancer Institute, this virus is spread by sharing syringes or needles, through blood transfusions or sexual contact, and from mother to child during birth or breast-feeding. Leukemia usually develops within a few decades of being infected, and it spreads rapidly, is essentially untreatable, and is almost always fatal.

> **"The American Cancer Society states that children and adults who undergo radiation therapy and/or chemotherapy have a higher risk of developing leukemia later in life, usually within 5 to 10 years of treatment."**

Another virus that has been connected with leukemia is the Epstein-Barr virus, which can contribute to the development of an aggressive form of lymphocytic leukemia known as Burkitt's leukemia. The Centers for Disease Control and Prevention states that this virus is a member of the herpes virus family and is one of the most common human viruses—an estimated 95 percent of adults between 35 and 40 years of age have been infected by it. Although most people who are infected with the Epstein-Barr virus never develop leukemia, it does increase their risk.

Leukemia Clusters

In February 2009 University of Arizona researchers Mark Witten and Paul Sheppard released a study that involved exposing mice to a highly toxic metal called tungsten. Tungsten is used in the manufacture of heavy tools for metalworking, oil and gas drilling, and other industries. After being exposed to tungsten, the mice developed leukemia-like symptoms and then became infected with a respiratory virus. Witten and Sheppard had been investigating the effects of tungsten since 2002, after 17 children from the small community of Fallon, Nevada, developed leukemia. Why such a large number of children had the disease was a mystery to scientists, although toxic substances in the environment had been suggested as a possible cause. A Centers for Disease Control and Prevention study published in 2003 showed that the urine samples of all the leukemia victims contained tungsten, and a report released the following year described the likelihood that environmental factors were involved. The report's authors wrote that "a cluster of this magnitude would be expected to occur in the United States by chance about once every 22,000 years," and went on to say that the Fallon leukemia outbreak "appears to be one of the most unusual childhood cancer clusters ever reported."[21]

> **"T-cell leukemia virus type 1, which is a distant cousin of the human immunovirus (HIV) that leads to AIDS, is linked to a very rare form of leukemia known as adult T-cell lymphocytic leukemia."**

During their investigation Witten and Sheppard studied tree rings in and around Fallon to gauge the amount of tungsten that had been deposited. "Trees take up metals from the environment and those metals show up in the tree rings," says Sheppard. "By analyzing chemicals in tree rings, we can look back in time years, and even decades."[22] The researchers found that the amount of tungsten had quadrupled between 1990 and 2002—and this was also the period of time in which all the children developed leukemia. Witten says that merits more research to determine the relationship between the disease and tungsten in the environment.

Another leukemia cluster has been identified in the region of Elbmarsch, Germany, and it is the largest cluster in the world. Between 1989 and 2009, 19 children from the area developed leukemia, a rate that is 3 or 4 times the country's average. Some German citizens are convinced that the outbreak resulted from a nuclear accident that occurred during the 1980s at the GKSS scientific research center and a fire that broke out at the Kruemmel nuclear power station, both of which are only a couple of miles from the town. Although officials connected with the 2 plants deny the connection between their facilities and the childhood leukemia cluster, a national survey performed at the end of 2007 showed that the risk of developing cancer rose dramatically for children who lived near a nuclear power plant. Uwe Harden, who is leading a citizens' group in Elbmarsch, shares his thoughts: "The figures are striking. It's not just a matter of chance. They tell us this is normal but they must think we're totally stupid."[23]

The Search Continues

Research has resulted in a number of likely contributors to leukemia, including hereditary factors, accompanying genetic disorders, exposure to environmental toxins, and viruses. Still, no one can say with any certainty what causes leukemia. It is especially puzzling to scientists because most people who have one or more risk factors never develop leukemia, while others with no risk factors *do* get it. Just as medical science has produced many answers about leukemia that were previously unknown, future research may reveal the exact cause or causes of the disease—and that could be the first step toward a cure.

Primary Source Quotes*

What Causes Leukemia?

"The cause of leukemia is not known. Chronic exposure to benzene in the workplace and exposure to extraordinary doses of irradiation can be causes of the disease, although neither explains most cases."

—Leukemia & Lymphoma Society, "Leukemia Facts & Statistics," June 17, 2009. www.leukemia-lymphoma.org.

Through blood research, education, and patient services, the Leukemia & Lymphoma Society seeks to cure leukemia, lymphoma, Hodgkin's disease, and myeloma and to improve the quality of life of patients and their families.

"Certain genetic diseases that cause children to be born with an abnormal immune system increase their risk of getting leukemia."

—American Cancer Society, "What Causes Childhood Leukemia?" May 15, 2009. www.cancer.org.

The American Cancer Society seeks to eliminate cancer as a major health problem by preventing it and saving lives through research, education, advocacy, and service.

---

* Editor's Note: While the definition of a primary source can be narrowly or broadly defined, for the purposes of Compact Research, a primary source consists of: 1) results of original research presented by an organization or researcher; 2) eyewitness accounts of events, personal experience, or work experience; 3) first-person editorials offering pundits' opinions; 4) government officials presenting political plans and/or policies; 5) representatives of organizations presenting testimony or policy.

"By now it is known that most patients have an anti-leukemia immune response. It remains a mystery as of why this immune response is incapable of providing a sufficient response to the disease."

—Doron Levy, "Leukemia Research," University of Maryland, June 2008. www.math.umd.edu.

Levy is a researcher and associate professor of mathematics at the University of Maryland.

"[Leukemia] cannot be passed on through contact nor through genes. There has been no evidence showing any hereditary connections."

—Leukemia Research Foundation, "Patient Information: FAQ," 2008. www.leukemia-research.org.

The mission of the Leukemia Research Foundation is to conquer leukemia and other blood cancers by funding research into their causes and cures and to enrich the life of those touched by the diseases.

"Doctors seldom know why one person gets leukemia and another doesn't. However, research shows that certain *risk factors* increase the chance that a person will get this disease."

—National Cancer Institute, "What You Need to Know About Leukemia," September 2008. www.cancer.gov.

The National Cancer Institute, which is an agency of the National Institutes of Health, is the U.S. government's principal federal agency for cancer research and training.

"Acute myelogenous leukemia appears to develop as a result of a defect in the immature cells of bone marrow."

—Cancer Treatment Centers of America, "Acute Myelogenous Leukemia—Prognosis," October 9, 2007. www.cancercenter.com.

The Cancer Treatment Centers of America is a cancer specialization medical facility that is committed to helping people overcome cancer.

"In most cases, neither parents nor children have control over the factors that trigger leukemia, although current studies are investigating the possibility that some environmental factors may predispose a child to develop the disease."

—Robin E. Miller, "Childhood Cancer: Leukemia," KidsHealth, June 2007. http://kidshealth.org.

Miller is a pediatrician in the division of hematology/oncology at Alfred I. duPont Hospital for Children in Wilmington, Delaware.

"The DNA of immature blood cells, mainly white cells, becomes damaged in some way. This abnormality causes the blood cells to grow and divide chaotically."

—Medical News Today, "What Is Leukemia? What Causes Leukemia?" March 17, 2009. www.medicalnewstoday.com.

With main offices in the United Kingdom, Medical News Today refers to itself as the largest independent health and medical news site on the Internet.

"Chronic lymphocytic leukemia is caused by damage to the DNA of newly forming cells in the bone marrow."

—Peter H. Gott, "Leukemia Causes Itchy Skin," *Park Hills (MO) Daily Journal*, October 20, 2008. www.dailyjournalonline.com.

Gott is a retired physician and the author of the book *Dr. Gott's No Flour, No Sugar Diet*.

What Causes Leukemia?

- The National Cancer Institute states that it is **rare for more than one person in a family to have leukemia**, and when it does happen, it most likely involves chronic lymphocytic leukemia.
- According to a Mayo Clinic researcher, if someone has a family member with chronic lymphocytic leukemia, his or her chances of getting the disease are **eight times higher** than that of the general population.
- Age is a significant factor in who develops certain types of leukemia; according to the Leukemia & Lymphoma Society, chronic lymphocytic leukemia incidence increases dramatically among people **50 years of age and older**, and acute myeloid leukemia incidence increases dramatically in people **55 and older.**
- Children have a **20 to 25 percent** chance of developing acute lymphocytic leukemia or acute myeloid leukemia if they have an identical twin who was diagnosed with the disease before the age of six.
- According to the National Down Syndrome Society, **1 in every 100 children** with Down syndrome develops leukemia, compared with **1 in every 2,000 children** who get the disease and do not have Down syndrome.
- Chronic myeloid leukemia is linked to a phenomenon called the **Philadelphia chromosome**, whereby pieces of chromosomes 9 and 22 break off and switch places.

Leukemia Risk Factors

Scientists do not know what causes leukemia—there is simply no explanation for why some people get the disease and others do not. Research has shown, however, that certain risk factors increase someone's chances of getting leukemia.

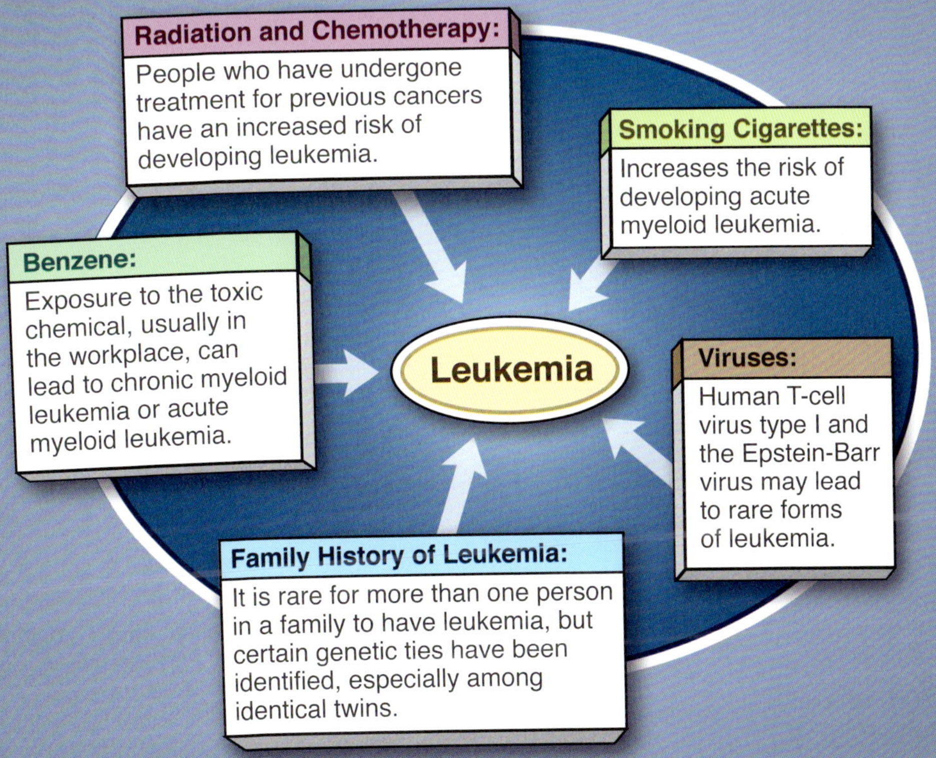

Source: National Cancer Institute, "What You Need to Know About Leukemia," September 2008.

- Race, combined with age, has been shown to be a factor in who develops leukemia; the Leukemia & Lymphoma Society states that **Hispanic children under the age of 20 have the highest rates of leukemia** of all races.

- The Epstein-Barr virus has been connected to an aggressive form of lymphocytic leukemia known as **Burkitt's leukemia**.

The Link Between Leukemia and Down Syndrome

Research has shown that children who are born with Down syndrome have a significantly higher likelihood of developing leukemia than children who do not have the disorder. This graph shows the comparison.

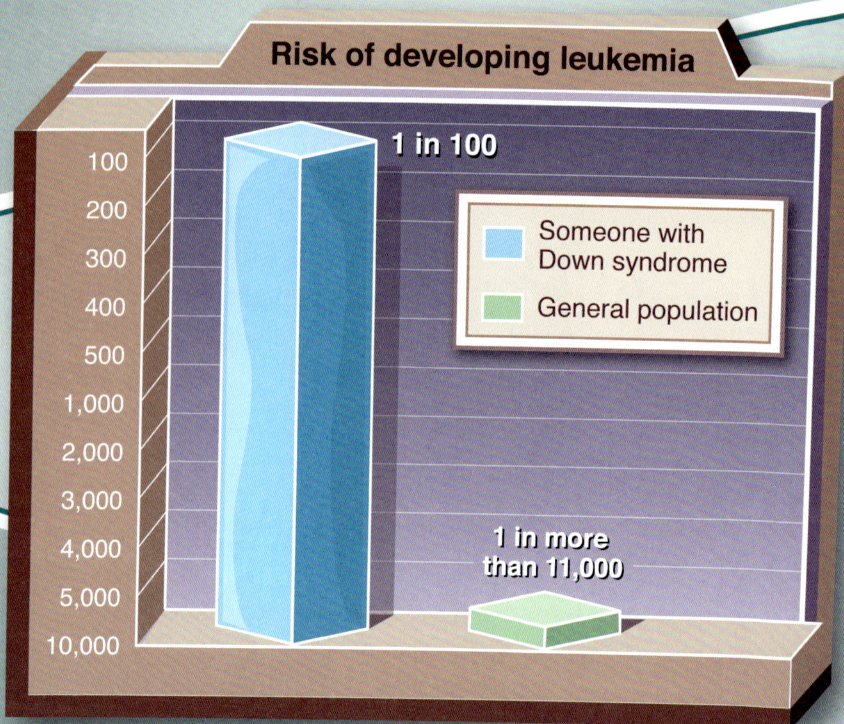

Sources: National Down Syndrome Society, "Down Syndrome Q & A: What Is Down Syndrome?" 2009. www.ndss.org; Aetna InteliHealth, "Leukemia," August 29, 2008. www.intelihealth.com.

- The University of California–San Francisco Medical Center states that **chromosomal abnormalities** are present in the majority of acute lymphocytic leukemia patients.

- Children with **Bloom's syndrome** and certain other genetic disorders have a higher risk of developing acute myeloid leukemia.

The Philadelphia Chromosome

Although scientists do not know why, they have discovered that people with chronic myeloid leukemia (CML) have an abnormal chromosome known as the Philadelphia chromosome. Every cell in the human body contains 23 pairs of chromosomes. The chromosomes are made up of DNA, which hold the instructions for the cells. The chromosomal abnormality forms when pieces of chromosomes 9 and 22 break off and exchange places. According to the Mayo Clinic, this creates an abnormally small chromosome 22 and a new combination of instructions for cells that can result in CML. This illustration shows how the Philadelphia chromosome forms.

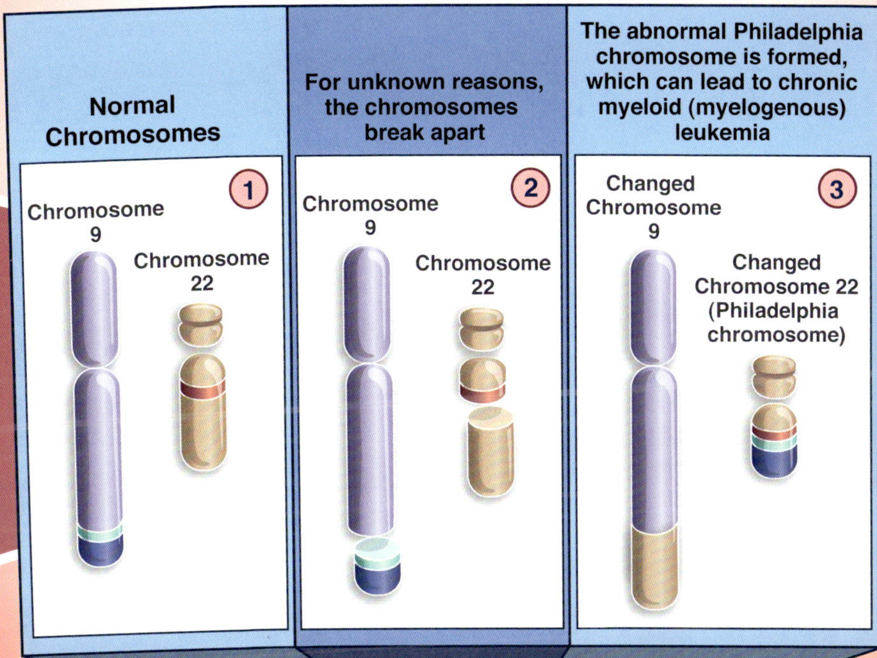

Sources: Mayo Clinic, "Chronic Myelogenous Leukemia: How the Philadelphia Chromosome Forms," June 23, 2009. www.mayoclinic.com.

- According to the American Cancer Society, survivors of the **atomic bomb explosions** in Japan in 1945 had a **20-fold increased risk of developing leukemia**, usually within 6 to 8 years after exposure.

How Successful Are Leukemia Treatments?

"The five-year relative survival rate has nearly quadrupled in the past 48 years for patients with leukemia."

—Leukemia & Lymphoma Society, which seeks to cure leukemia and improve the quality of life of patients and their families through research, education, and patient services.

"Most childhood leukemias have very high remission rates. And the majority of children can be cured—meaning that they are in permanent remission—of the disease."

—Robin E. Miller, a hematology/oncology pediatrician at Alfred I. duPont Hospital for Children in Wilmington, Delaware.

On November 13, 2008, Mandy and Rob Garola heard something from a pediatrician that is every parent's worst nightmare—it was very likely that their little daughter had cancer. Two-year-old Cora had been suffering from constant ear infections, she was pale and tired all the time, and she was exhibiting grouchy behavior that was not typical for her. After a series of blood tests, the pediatrician suspected leukemia and advised the Garolas to take Cora to the hospital, where she was diagnosed with acute lymphocytic leukemia (ALL). As stricken as they were over hearing about their daughter's disease, they were relieved when doctors told them that of all forms of leukemia, ALL was the best one to have because most children who undergo treatment are cured. Over the following months, Cora was in and out of the hospital. She underwent 3 blood transfusions, 1 platelet transfusion, chemotherapy, and several bone marrow procedures, and as of May 2009 she was in remission. "Thirty years ago, leukemia was a death sentence," says Mandy Garola. "It's not now."[24]

Chemotherapy Treatments

One of the most common treatments for leukemia is chemotherapy, whereby cancer-killing drugs are injected into a muscle or vein or are given orally in the form of a pill. Because leukemic cells divide and reproduce constantly, the goal of chemotherapy is to kill all rapidly dividing cells in the body—which means it also kills healthy blood cells. This often results in side effects such as nausea, diarrhea or constipation, sores in the mouth, and loss of body and scalp hair.

Donnie Wilemon was plagued with unpleasant side effects after being treated with chemotherapy. Diagnosed with acute myeloid leukemia in March 2004, Wilemon was in his thirties and otherwise in good health, so his physician thought he had a very good chance of beating the cancer with chemotherapy only, rather than a combination of treatments. He describes his first experience with chemotherapy and what he went through afterward:

> I watched as the "Drain-O" slowly descended into my body, almost expecting some sort of instantaneous reaction. Somewhat anticlimactic, nothing really happened to me physically for a couple of days—I remember commenting that it wasn't any "big deal." Little did I know that it takes a couple of days for the chemo to take full effect—it starts with gradual impact . . . but sometime around the third day the massive, cumulative impact of the chemotherapy hit me almost at once. My blood numbers dropped dramatically almost overnight. I felt like I had the worst stomach-virus of my entire life. I can not adequately explain in words how profoundly lifeless and tired I became during this time.[25]

Wilemon says that his misery did not last for long, and within a few days he began to feel much better. As of June 2009 his leukemia was still in remission after 5 years.

The Pros and Cons of Radiation Therapy

When leukemic cells are located in areas of the body that chemotherapy cannot reach (such as around the brain and spinal cord), patients may undergo radiation therapy. This treatment utilizes highly complex machines that are the same type used for diagnostic X-rays, but deliver much higher doses of radiation to specific places in the body. One type, known as external beam radiation, is used most often to treat people with leukemia or other blood cancers. According to the Leukemia & Lymphoma Society, the procedure involves focusing a beam of radiation on the outside of the patient's body by a machine called a linear accelerator, which can move around to deliver radiation from various angles. Radiation therapy kills cancer cells and also damages some healthy cells, but the damaged cells usually recover and return to normal functioning after treatment is stopped. There are risks involved with radiation, however, especially for children. It has been shown to contribute to other cancers later in life, as well as stunted growth, hormonal imbalances, and cognitive deficits such as learning disabilities.

> **"One of the most common treatments for leukemia is chemotherapy, whereby cancer-killing drugs are injected into a muscle or vein or are given orally in the form of a pill."**

At St. Jude Children's Research Hospital, radiation therapy had long been the standard treatment for children with ALL in order to prevent the leukemia from spreading to the central nervous system. But because of the damaging side effects, radiation dosages were steadily reduced over the years, and radiation therapy was limited to only the highest-risk patients. In June 2009 St. Jude researchers announced the results of a study that involved 498 children who were treated for ALL between 2000 and 2007. In order to analyze the effectiveness of radiation treatments versus chemotherapy in reducing the relapse rate, the researchers compared the outcomes of 71 patients whose leukemias would have qualified them for radiation with the outcomes of 56 patients who had been treated with radiation therapy in the past. The result was that the 71 patients had markedly better remission rates than the 56 patients who had been treated with radiation. This finding convinced the researchers that radiation could be safely eliminated in all patients by substituting personalized chemotherapy regimens. "The bottom line is that not only did we get outstanding treatment responses in these patients, many of whom would have otherwise received irradiation, but they will have a better quality of life because of the absence of its side effects,"[26] says St. Jude cancer specialist Dr. Ching-Hon Pui.

Biological Therapy

Because of the many side effects that are associated with chemotherapy and radiation, researchers have been investigating treatments that could be just as effective but less harsh for leukemia patients. A fairly new type of treatment is known as biological therapy, which is also called immunotherapy. Biological therapy uses the body's immune system to fight leukemia.

In order to understand how this treatment works, it is important to know how vital the immune system is to the body, as well as the functions it performs. A complex collection of organs, tissues, and cells, the immune system protects the body against millions of bacteria, viruses, toxins, and parasites. HowStuffWorks founder Marshall Brain explains its importance:

> When something dies, its immune system (along with everything else) shuts down. In a matter of hours, the body is invaded by all sorts of bacteria, microbes, parasites. . . . None of these things are able to get in when your immune system is working, but the moment your immune system stops the door is wide open. Once you die it only takes a few weeks for these organisms to completely dismantle your body and carry it away, until all that's left is a skeleton. Obviously your immune system is doing something amazing to keep all of that dismantling from happening when you are alive.[27]

Although scientists are not certain how the immune system protects against cancer, it is likely that it recognizes the difference between healthy cells and cancerous cells in the body and works to eliminate those that become cancerous.

In someone with leukemia, the immune system's function is impaired because of the proliferation of abnormal white blood cells in the bloodstream. Biological therapies are designed to repair, stimulate, and/or enhance the immune system's responses when cancerous cells prevent it from functioning correctly. The Leukemia & Lymphoma Society says the theory behind immunotherapy is that immune cells can be engineered to recognize and kill cancerous cells. For instance, one type involves the production of monoclonal antibodies, which are proteins produced in the laboratory that are designed to target and destroy cells by recognizing specific structures (antigens) on their surface. This sort of treatment is administered to the patient by intravenous infusion, during which each monoclonal antibody is designed to bind to a specific antigen on a cancer cell and rid the body of the abnormal cells. According to Patricia Keegan, who is with the U.S. Food and Drug Administration's Center for Biologics Evaluation and Research, biological therapy can be effective in treating different types of leukemia. She adds, however, that there are few laboratory-produced therapies available because "they are labor-intensive—the development of blood products is a relatively young field that is still developing."[28]

> **"This finding convinced the researchers that radiation could be safely eliminated in all patients by substituting personalized chemotherapy regimens."**

Replacing Cancerous Blood with Healthy Blood

In 1956 New York physician E. Donnall Thomas made medical history when he performed the world's first bone marrow transplant and in the process, saved a young leukemia patient's life. At the time such procedures were unheard of, and scientists were not sure what it was about bone marrow that had healing properties. Years later it was discovered that stem cells produced within marrow had the ability to enter the bloodstream of the patient and begin destroying cancerous cells as they produced healthy blood cells.

Today bone marrow transplants (often called stem cell transplants) have proved to be successful in curing a number of leukemia sufferers. The patient first receives intense chemotherapy, and sometimes radiation therapy, to destroy cancerous cells in the bone marrow. After stem cells have been harvested (either from a donor or from the patient when he or she was in remission), they are administered through a catheter that is inserted into a large vein. If the procedure is successful, new blood cells begin to grow from the transplanted stem cells and replace those that were destroyed.

When Treatments Fail

Over the years many treatments have been developed that now give leukemia sufferers a better chance than ever of beating their disease. According to the Leukemia & Lymphoma Society, the survival rate has improved dramatically in the past 4 decades, as it writes: "In 1960–63, when compared to a person without leukemia, a patient had a 14 percent chance of living five years. By 1975–1977, the five year relative survival rate had jumped to 35 percent, and in 1996–2004 the overall relative survival rate was slightly above 50 percent."[29] The organization adds that the survival rate for CLL is now 76.2 percent, and for ALL is 66.1 percent for adults and 91.2 percent for children younger than 5 years old. Yet even with all the progress that has been made, leukemia remains a disease that kills. The Leukemia & Lymphoma Society states that it claims the lives of more than 21,000 people in the United States each year, and it is the fifth most common cause of cancer deaths.

> **"Biological therapies are designed to repair, stimulate, and/or enhance the immune system's responses when cancerous cells prevent it from functioning correctly."**

One person who underwent comprehensive treatments but lost his battle with leukemia was Blake LaForce, an 18-year-old former high school football star from Vandalia, Ohio. After being diagnosed with ALL in November 2007, LaForce underwent a bone marrow transplant the following May. A month later tests showed that his body had accepted the transplanted stem cells and there were no longer any leukemia cells, which was excellent news for him and his family. But in mid-August LaForce developed a devastating infection of the nervous system that rendered him unable to walk, talk, eat, or drink. Even then, he seemed to be slowly getting better, until March 26, 2009, when he suffered a pulmonary hemorrhage (bleeding lungs), and later developed a severe skin problem. In a July 2, 2009, post in an online journal, Blake LaForce's father described his son's condition: "Blake's skin is almost like a burn victim's skin now, so the risk of infection increases. It is another one of God's miracles because Blake is actually very stable and not even on any pain medications, which is unbelievable. There are what seems an endless number of hurdles on Blake's journey and we are in awe of his stamina, true grit and resolve."[30] In spite of managing to fight his long battle with leukemia, however, LaForce died 2 days after his father's post.

> **"Even with all the progress that has been made, leukemia remains a disease that kills."**

Hope for Tomorrow

No treatment is guaranteed to cure leukemia, and thousands of people still die from it each year. But scientists have made outstanding progress in developing chemotherapy methods and other treatments that have vastly improved survival rates and offer those who suffer from leukemia more hope than ever before. With future research, and the inevitable progress that will be made, the likelihood that leukemia will eventually be conquered becomes more realistic each day.

Primary Source Quotes*

How Successful Are Leukemia Treatments?

"For some types of childhood cancer, the improvements have been mind boggling—acute lymphoblastic leukemia (the most common type of cancer in children) has changed from a disease that killed almost everyone who contracted it within 3 months, to a disease that is cured 75% of the time."

—David Loeb, "September Is National Childhood Cancer Awareness Month," Dr. David's Blog, September 15, 2008. http://doctordavidsblog.blogspot.com.

Loeb is a pediatric oncologist (cancer specialist) from Baltimore, Maryland.

"Unlike other types of cancer, leukemia isn't a solid tumor that your doctor can surgically remove. Leukemia treatment is complex."

—Mayo Clinic, "Leukemia," April 5, 2008. www.mayoclinic.com.

The Mayo Clinic is a world-renowned medical practice that is dedicated to the diagnosis and treatment of virtually every type of complex illness.

* Editor's Note: While the definition of a primary source can be narrowly or broadly defined, for the purposes of Compact Research, a primary source consists of: 1) results of original research presented by an organization or researcher, 2) eyewitness accounts of events, personal experience, or work experience; 3) first-person editorials offering pundits' opinions; 4) government officials presenting political plans and/or policies; 5) representatives of organizations presenting testimony or policy.

"Forty years ago, ALL was incurable. Today, in the United States, its cure rate is a major success story—as many as 90 percent of the kids who have it are cured. But worldwide, ALL remains the leading cancer-killer of children."

—National Institutes of Health, "Curing Children's Cancer," *MedLine Plus*, Summer 2008. www.nlm.nih.gov.

The National Institutes of Health is the United States' primary agency for conducting and supporting medical research.

"Hairy-cell leukemia is a relatively rare form of adult chronic leukemia. . . . This disease was once uniformly fatal, but highly successful therapies have been developed, and patients today who receive proper treatment can have a relatively normal quality of life."

—Ohio State University Comprehensive Cancer Center-James Cancer Hospital and Solove Research Institute, "50 Years of Hairy-Cell Leukemia to Be Observed," December 4, 2008. http://medicalcenter.osu.edu.

Ohio State University Comprehensive Cancer Center-James Cancer Hospital and Solove Research Institute is one of 40 National Cancer Institute–designated comprehensive cancer centers in the United States and the only freestanding cancer hospital in the Midwest.

"Many people with acute leukemia can be cured. . . . Chronic leukemia can seldom be cured."

—National Institutes of Health, "X-Plain Leukemia: Reference Summary," April 16, 2008. www.nlm.nih.gov.

The National Institutes of Health is the United States' primary agency for conducting and supporting medical research.

"Just 50 years ago, the diagnosis of acute leukemia was a death warrant. Patients looked forward to an immediate onset of bleeding from mouth, nose, urine, rectum, major infection, and a lifespan of approximately two months on average, with virtually 100% mortality by one year after diagnosis."

—Emil J. Freireich, "A Word on Leukemia and Progress from Dr. Emil J.," Accelerate Progress, 2009. http://accelerateprogress.org.

Freireich is a physician who specializes in cancer and is a past president of the American Society of Clinical Oncologists.

"This form of leukemia [caused by an abnormality of the MLL gene] in infants and children has a very poor outcome with therapy. I want to change that."

—John H. Kersey, "Meet the Researchers Conducting Breakthrough Research," Children's Cancer Research Fund, 2009. www.childrenscancer.org.

Kersey is a pediatric cancer specialist and professor at the University of Minnesota Departments of Laboratory Medicine/Pathology and Pediatrics.

"Unfortunately, the prognosis for JMML [juvenile myelomonocytic leukemia] is very poor. In general, the children do not respond to standard chemotherapy that would be used for regular infant leukemia. Most of the cases are fatal by the time the child is 3 years old."

—Gary Kleiner, "In-Depth Interview: Stem Cells Help Kids with Cancer," WCTV interview, December 26, 2008. www.wctv.tv.

Kleiner is an associate professor of clinical pediatrics and an assistant professor of surgery at the University of Miami Leonard M. Miller School of Medicine.

"Despite radiation's success in treating [acute lymphoblastic leukemia], it produces side effects that include second cancers, stunted growth, hormone imbalances and cognitive deficits."

—St. Jude Children's Research Hospital, "St. Jude Study Shows Personalized Chemotherapy Can Improve Cure Rate and Avoid the Use of Radiation in Acute Lymphoblastic Leukemia Treatment," June 24, 2009. www.stjude.org.

St. Jude Children's Research Hospital is a renowned pediatric treatment and research facility located in Memphis, Tennessee.

How Successful Are Leukemia Treatments?

- According to the American Cancer Society, death rates from leukemia in males and females combined have decreased by about **1.5 percent** per year since 2000.

- The 5-year survival rate for children under the age of 15 who have acute lymphocytic leukemia rose from **3 percent** in 1964 to nearly **90 percent** in 2004.

- A 2009 report by the Leukemia & Lymphoma Society states that in the early 1960s, a patient with leukemia only had a **14 percent** chance of living 5 years, compared with today, when the average survival rate is **51 percent**.

- The average survival rate for patients with chronic lymphocytic leukemia is nearly **79 percent**.

- According to the Leukemia & Lymphoma Society, a drug known as cladribine has been shown to result in long-term remissions in nearly **90 percent** of patients treated within one week of being diagnosed with hairy cell leukemia.

- The American Association for Cancer Research states that **radiation therapy** is most commonly used to target high percentages of leukemia cells gathered in specific regions of the body, such as the brain or cerebrospinal fluid.

A Dramatic Improvement in Survival Rates Among Children

Decades ago children who were diagnosed with leukemia faced certain death—the disease was considered incurable and was always fatal. Thanks to scientific research, which has produced many successful treatments, a diagnosis of leukemia today is not necessarily a death sentence. This graph shows how the survival rate for children has increased since the 1960s.

Five-year survival rates for children with acute lymphocytic leukemia

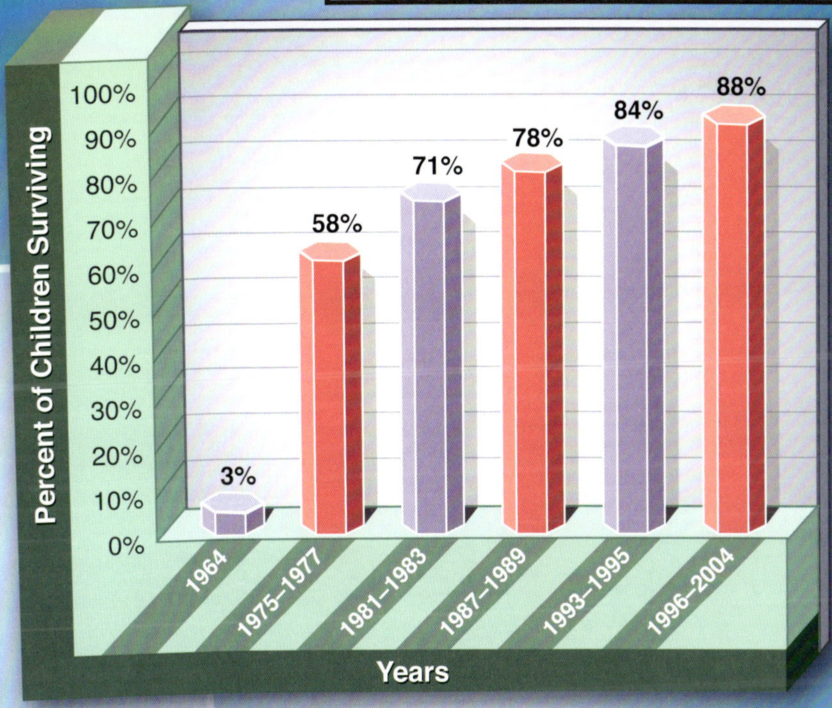

Source: Leukemia & Lymphoma Society, "Leukemia Facts & Statistics," July 1, 2009. www.leukemia-lymphoma.org.

- The Leukemia & Lymphoma Society states that there are approximately **50 different chemotherapeutic agents** used to treat patients with leukemia and other blood cancers.

Survival Rates for Leukemia Versus Other Cancers

According to the Leukemia & Lymphoma Society, the survival rate for people diagnosed with leukemia has nearly quadrupled since 1960. Experts credit improved treatments for this change. This graph shows how leukemia survival rates are better than some types of cancer but still worse than others.

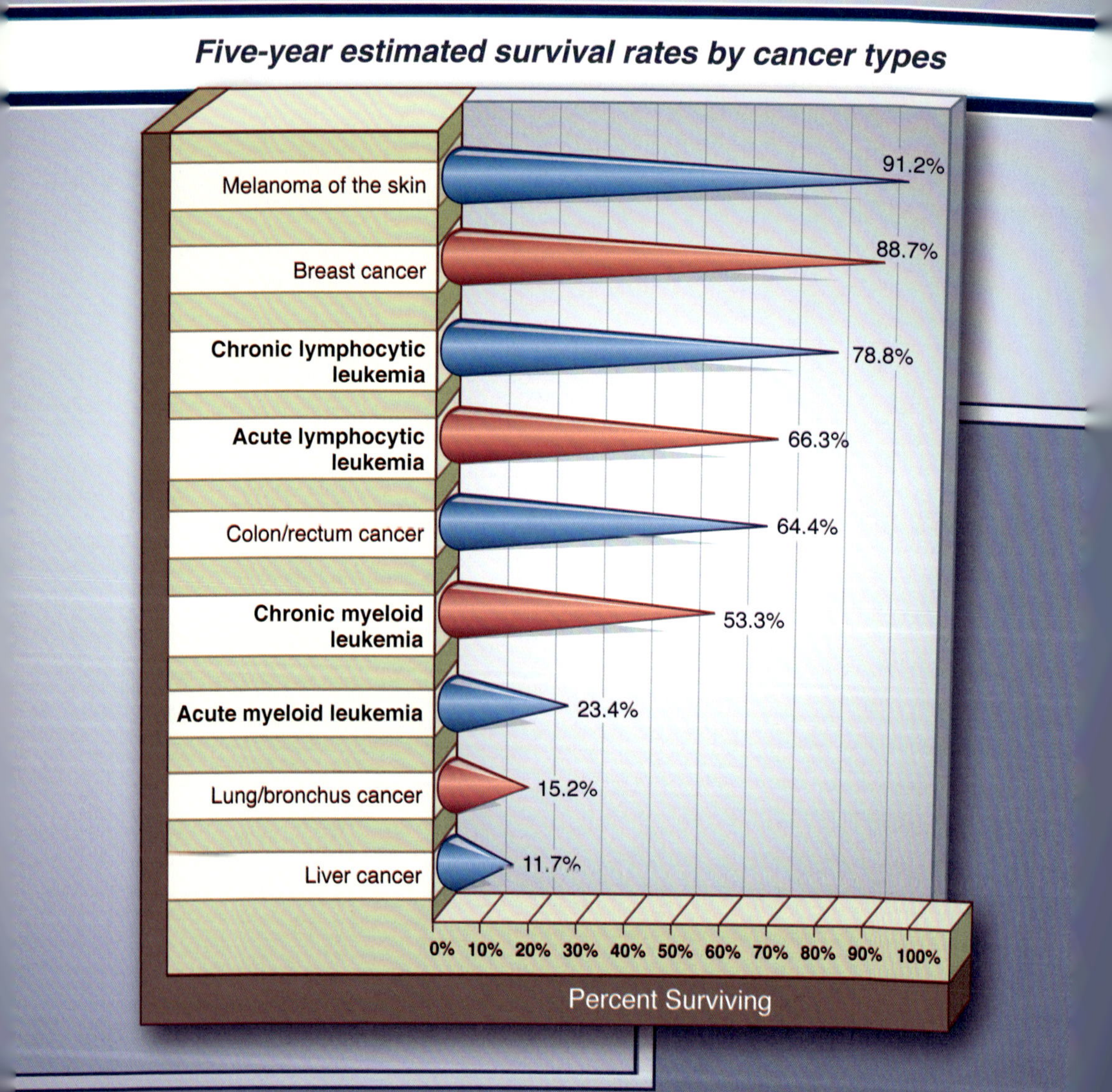

Sources: American Cancer Society, "Cancer Facts & Figures 2009," 2009. www.cancer.org; Leukemia & Lymphoma Society, "Leukemia Facts & Statistics," July 1, 2009. www.leukemia-lymphoma.org.

Leukemia Can Still Be Deadly

Even though chemotherapy and other treatments have made it possible for many leukemia patients to beat their disease and live long, cancer-free lives, leukemia is still the fifth most common cause of cancer deaths in the United States, as this graph illustrates.

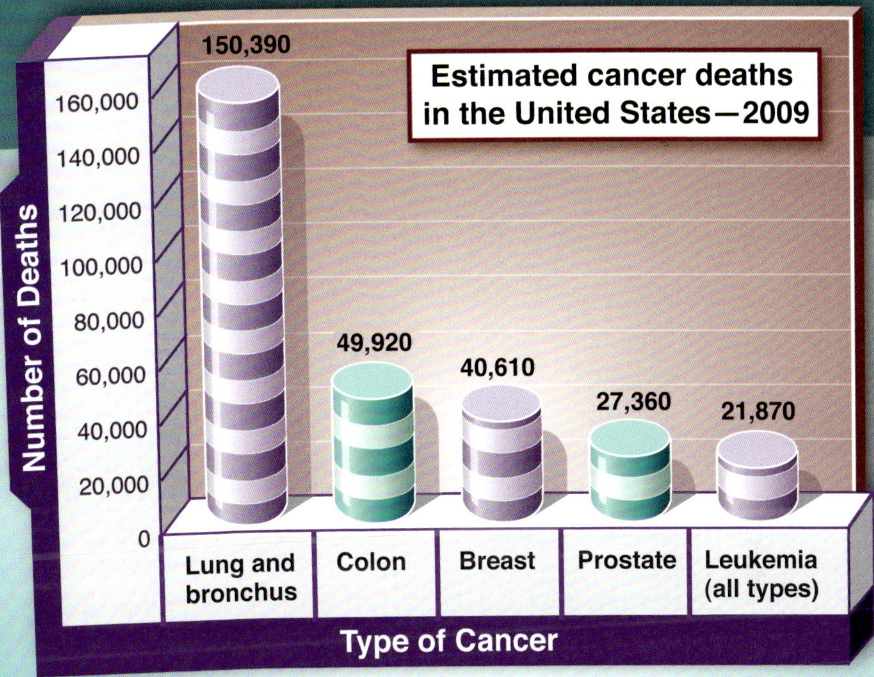

Source: American Cancer Society, "Cancer Facts & Figures 2009," 2009. www.cancer.org.

- Between 2001 and 2005 **African Americans** between the ages of 25 and 64 with leukemia had a higher death rate than Caucasians who were diagnosed with the disease.

- Patients who are considered the **best candidates for stem cell transplants** are those who have the fast-growing forms of leukemia, are younger than age 55, and have a relative who is an identical match and can be a bone marrow donor.

What Are the Prospects for Preventing or Curing Leukemia?

"The research being done today will save the children of tomorrow."

—Julie Ross, the director of the division of pediatric epidemiology and clinical research at the University of Minnesota.

"Thanks to scientific progress, we've seen a dramatic improvement in childhood cancer survival rates since the 1960s. Back then, only a quarter of kids survived cancer, compared with three-quarters who survive today."

—Cancer Research UK, which is one of the world's leading independent organizations dedicated to cancer research.

Rudolph and Antoinette de Villiers were heartbroken when their 16-year-old son died from leukemia in 1944. At that time the diagnosis was devastating because it meant certain death—no one survived the disease. Five years later the New York couple was still frustrated because there were no treatments available to help others who suffered from leukemia, so they decided to do something about it. In 1949, with only a few willing volunteers, a small office, and a minuscule budget, the de Villiers started a fund-raising and education organization in their son's name, the Robert Roesler de Villiers Foundation. They were well aware that the task they faced was daunting because leukemia was totally mystifying to scientists. Most leukemia patients, especially children, only lived about 3 months after being diagnosed, and the disease was considered incurable. Even by the mid-1950s, when the first chemotherapy drugs started to become available, leukemia remained a killer, as the foundation's 1955 annual report stated: "As of this date, Leukemia is 100% fatal. This is almost a unique situation among the many diseases to which man is susceptible."[31]

Over the years the de Villiers's foundation steadily grew, raised hundreds of millions of dollars, and changed its name several times, to the Leukemia Society, the Leukemia Society of America, and finally the Leukemia & Lymphoma Society, which it is known as today. Since its first funding in 1954, the organization has awarded more than $600 million for research on leukemia and other blood cancers, and it has financially supported numerous researchers who have developed lifesaving leukemia treatments. These monies, along with funds generated by other private organizations and funding from federal sources, have resulted in leukemia no longer being a disease that always claims the lives of its victims. Today, because of amazing scientific progress, leukemia sufferers have one thing that did not exist decades ago: hope.

"Of all the types of leukemia that have been identified, by far, acute myeloid leukemia (AML) has the poorest prognosis."

A Promising Discovery

Of all the types of leukemia that have been identified, by far, acute myeloid leukemia (AML) has the poorest prognosis. Survival rates for the disease are grim: only 21 percent overall, and 55 percent for children who are diagnosed before the age of 15. Although scientists have learned that AML does not respond well to chemotherapy and has a high relapse rate, the reasons for this are not known. "The cellular and molecular basis for this dismal picture is unclear," says Richard Lock, a researcher with the Children's Cancer Institute Australia and the University of New South Wales. "However, previous research has suggested that leukemia stem cells (LSCs) may lie at the heart of post-treatment relapse and chemoresistance."[32] Because of a study announced in July 2009 by Lock and his team of researchers, the outlook for people with AML may improve dramatically.

The researchers had observed that a particular molecule exists at very high levels on leukemia stem cells but not on normal blood cells. The molecule plays an important role in regulating the body's immunity, as well as inducing the process by which stem cells evolve into different types of blood cells. Because the molecule was abundant only in leukemia stem cells, the researchers suspected that its presence was linked to the uncontrolled production of abnormal white blood cells in bone marrow, the hallmark of leukemia. Following this theory, they created an antibody that was designed to bind to the molecule in the hope that it would interfere with the survival and growth of cancerous cells.

> **"In addition to paving the way to improved treatments, the study could potentially lead to methods of perfecting bone marrow transplants that could boost the chance that patients can be cured of leukemia."**

After treating mice with the antibody, the researchers injected the creatures with leukemia stem cells that were taken from blood samples of AML patients—and the results proved to be remarkable. As planned, the antibody bound to the abnormal cells. It then blocked the production of leukemia cells, prohibited existing leukemia cells from traveling through the bloodstream to bone marrow, and boosted the immune systems of the mice so the leukemia cells were destroyed. Overall, treatment with the antibody vastly improved mouse survival when compared with a control group of mice that had not been treated with it. Because the experiment yielded such promising findings, Locke and his team of researchers began clinical trials with human patients shortly afterward. They are convinced that their discovery holds immense potential for the development of future treatments for AML as well as other cancers.

Identifying a Key Gene

Scientists have long suspected that genetic mutations play at least some role in who develops leukemia and who does not—and in April 2009 a team from the University of California–San Francisco announced a study that confirmed it. The team, led by Emmanuelle Passegué, discovered that a gene known as JunB plays a key role in controlling the rapid production of stem cells in the body, as well as determines what types of blood cells they differentiate into. The researchers studied the behavior of stem cells that were deficient in JunB, both in culture dishes and when transplanted into mice. In every case they found that the JunB-deficient stem cells led to the development of a disorder that causes stem cells to become cancerous and is a precursor to leukemia.

> **"In December 2008 the team announced that when they exposed leukemia cells to high doses of [grape seed] extract, this triggered the death of 76 percent of the cancerous cells, yet the procedure did not harm normal cells."**

This led to their conclusion that leukemia is caused by a proliferation of JunB-deficient stem cells in the bloodstream, which allows the overproduction of abnormal cells. Passegué explains the significance of this discovery: "By uncovering this mechanism, we might one day be able to determine the difference between normal [stem cells] and leukemic stem cells. . . . This could allow us to develop more targeted therapies. These kinds of therapeutic applications are still down the road, but they can happen very quickly in the blood/leukemia field."[33] In addition to paving the way to improved treatments, the study could potentially lead to methods of perfecting bone marrow transplants that could boost the chance that patients can be cured of leukemia.

Green Tea and Grape Seeds

People in Asian countries such as China and Japan have a significantly lower risk of developing cancer than those who live in Western countries. This is not well understood, although a major theory is that their diets, which are much lower in fat than the typical American diet, play an important role in the low cancer rates. Another theory involves green tea. In China, Japan, and other parts of Asia, people traditionally drink green tea. The beverage contains high levels of epigallocatechin gallate (EGCG), a natural chemical that is believed to be an anticarcinogen. Although green tea has long been studied as a substance that could contribute to improved health, the possibility that it could be used to cure disease has seldom been investigated. That will likely change based on a May 2009 announcement by researchers at the Mayo Clinic.

Using blood samples from patients with chronic lymphocytic leukemia, researcher Kit Lee added EGCG to the blood in test tubes and found that 80 percent of the blood cells showed improvement. Follow-up clinical trials with laboratory animals produced similar results, so the next step was human clinical trials. In May 2009 the Mayo Clinic team reported that the participants had responded well to high doses of EGCG (given in capsule form), and one-third of them saw a reduction in leukemia blood cells. The hope is that this will lead to a new type of therapy for CLL patients that is as effective (or even more effective) in fighting the disease but without the harsh side effects of chemotherapy.

> **With all the progress that has been made over the years, and the innumerable scientific achievements, the future looks brighter than ever before for people who are diagnosed with leukemia.**

Another experimental leukemia treatment is also derived from a natural source: grape seeds. As a December 2008 article on Medical News Today explains: "An extract from grape seeds forces laboratory leukemia cells to commit cell suicide."[34] Laboratory studies have shown that grape seed extract, which is commercially available, may be effective in treating malignant cells, including those that result in skin, breast, colon, lung, stomach, or prostate cancers. The substance had never been used on leukemia cells until researchers from the University of Kentucky began experiments with grape seed extract. In December 2008 the team announced that when they exposed leukemia cells to high doses of the extract, the procedure triggered the death of 76 percent of the cancerous cells but did not harm normal cells. The scientists are hopeful that this discovery will lead to treatments that kill leukemia cells in the bloodstream but, unlike chemotherapy and radiation therapy, leave healthy cells alone.

The Miracle Inside Sponges

Since 1995 scientists have known about the anti-leukemia potential of kapakahines, natural products that are derived from marine sponges and have proved to be toxic to cancerous cells. The tube-shaped sponges, known as *Cribrochalina olemda*, are found on reefs throughout many tropical areas of the world, such as in the South Pacific. They naturally produce a molecule called kapakahine B, which has shown potential for fighting leukemia. But because each sponge contains no more than a speck of kapakahines, researchers had not been able to amass a significant enough quantity to conduct any meaningful studies. Scientists throughout the world tried to replicate the substances without success. "Chemists are always attracted to things that are bizarre," says Phil Baran, a scientist at the Scripps Research Institute. "There is no shortage of biologists who want to look at active molecules, but if you can't provide the molecule, then they can't go very far."[35]

Finally, in April 2009 Baran and a team of Scripps researchers announced that they had succeeded where others had failed, and had synthesized kapakahines in large quantities in their laboratory. That is an exciting development because, for the first time, full research into the compounds' potential can begin and may eventually lead to the development of drugs that can prevent or treat leukemia and other forms of cancer.

Overcoming Drug Resistance

Once considered a leading killer of children, acute lymphocytic leukemia now has a survival rate of more than 90 percent among those who are diagnosed and treated before the age of five. But many children who do not survive ALL are resistant to chemotherapy and/or develop allergic reactions to drugs, meaning that treatment may not be possible for them. This has long been puzzling and frustrating for scientists, but a study released in June 2009 may have helped solve the mystery.

Researchers in the United Kingdom identified an enzyme that is responsible for breaking down and inactivating an anticancer drug commonly used to treat young ALL sufferers. The researchers found that the enzyme breaks the drug down in the bloodstream and in the process prevents it from working properly. "Although our results are at an early stage," says researcher Vaskar Saha, "our study is an important development in understanding the science behind why some patients don't respond to leukaemia drugs. If our findings in leukaemia cells are confirmed in patients, we could be able to test if this drug is the best option before treatment starts."[36] Many scientists are enthusiastic about the finding because it offers an explanation of how and why resistance to the drug occurs and opens up the possibility of modifying the drug so patients are able to overcome the resistance.

Looking Toward the Future

Leukemia research has come an amazingly long way since the 1950s, when the disease was considered incurable and everyone who developed it was expected to die. Scientists are constantly making new discoveries about genes, proteins, cells, and enzymes that play key roles in who develops leukemia and who does not. Their findings have led to promising new treatments that offer leukemia patients hope that they never dared to have in the past. With all the progress that has been made over the years and the innumerable scientific achievements, the future looks brighter than ever before for people who are diagnosed with leukemia. No one can say for sure, but there may come a time when the disease is talked about as nothing more than a thing of the past.

Primary Source Quotes*

What Are the Prospects for Preventing or Curing Leukemia?

"In the next few years, I think there will be . . . exciting developments in leukemia genetics and genetics as a whole."

—Ross L. Levine, "An Interview with Ross L. Levine," Memorial Sloan-Kettering Cancer Center interview, March 2009. www.mskcc.org.

Levine is an oncologist with Memorial Sloan-Kettering Cancer Center in New York City.

"Pediatric cancer research is at a pivotal junction. Breakthroughs are being discovered at increasing frequency."

—John E. Wagner, "Meet the Researchers Conducting Breakthrough Research," Children's Cancer Research Fund, 2009. www.childrenscancer.org.

Wagner is professor of pediatrics and director of the division of hematology-oncology and blood and marrow transplantation at the University of Minnesota.

* Editor's Note: While the definition of a primary source can be narrowly or broadly defined, for the purposes of Compact Research, a primary source consists of: 1) results of original research presented by an organization or researcher; 2) eyewitness accounts of events, personal experience, or work experience; 3) first-person editorials offering pundits' opinions; 4) government officials presenting political plans and/or policies; 5) representatives of organizations presenting testimony or policy.

"The last 30 years of cancer 'progress' have failed the next generation of survivors so there is no reason to think the next 30 will be any different unless change happens now."

—I'm Too Young for This! Cancer Research, "Stupid Cancer 101," 2009. http://i2y.com.

The goal of I'm Too Young for This! Cancer Research is to increase the five-year survival rate for young adults while empowering them to achieve their peak potential.

"The development of new drugs and combinations of drugs that target particular proteins found in leukemia cells continues to be a major area of research and discovery."

—American Association for Cancer Research, "Leukemia," June 23, 2008. www.aacr.org.

The American Association for Cancer Research's mission is to prevent and cure cancer through research, education, communication, and collaboration.

"Research on the causes, diagnosis, and treatment of acute leukemia is being done at many world-renowned cancer research centers."

—American Cancer Society, "What's New in Adult Acute Leukemia Research and Treatment?" 2009. www.cancer.org.

The American Cancer Society seeks to eliminate cancer as a major health problem by preventing it and saving lives through research, education, advocacy, and service.

"Scientists are studying ways to boost the body's natural defenses, called immunotherapy. The goal is to kill or prevent the growth of [leukemia] cells."

—Leukemia & Lymphoma Society, "Acute Myelogenous Leukemia," June 17, 2009. www.leukemia-lymphoma.org.

The Leukemia & Lymphoma Society seeks to cure leukemia, lymphoma, Hodgkin's disease, and myeloma and to improve the quality of life of patients and their families.

"By growing leukemia cells in mice and giving them various forms of antibodies, immune cells, or chemotherapeutic drugs, we can study ways to treat the difficult MLL-AF4 [genetic-based] leukemia. Laboratory research should help us better predict which treatments may be more effective for children suffering from . . . infant leukemia."

—John H. Kersey, "Pursuing a Better Understanding of Childhood Leukemia," Children's Cancer Research Fund, 2009. www.childrenscancer.org.

Kersey is a pediatric cancer specialist and a professor at the University of Minnesota Departments of Laboratory Medicine/Pathology and Pediatrics.

"Further research can ultimately translate into safer and more effective methods of treating our patients with leukemia."

—Children's Cancer Research Fund, "Double Umbilical Cord Blood Transplantation Offers Promise for Leukemia Patients," 2009. www.childrenscancer.org.

The Children's Cancer Research Fund is dedicated to finding a cure for childhood cancer by providing funds to the University of Minnesota for research and training relating to the prevention, treatment, and cure of childhood cancer.

What Are the Prospects for Preventing or Curing Leukemia?

- According to the American Cancer Society, scientists have made much progress in understanding how **changes in a person's DNA can cause normal bone marrow cells to develop into leukemia**, and the hope is that this will lead to the development of new targeted therapies.

- Despite the fact that survival rates have improved dramatically, leukemia still causes **more deaths among children and young adults under the age of 20** than any other cancer.

- Studies have shown that adult survivors of acute lymphocytic leukemia are at high risk for developing **osteoporosis or other diseases** (likely caused by chemotherapy and other treatments), so a major focus of new research is on the long-term effects of these treatments.

- Researchers are closely studying whether **cancer vaccines** used to boost the immune system would be effective in fighting leukemia cells in the body.

- According to the American Cancer Society, researchers have developed a test called **PCR that can find one leukemia cell among a million normal** cells, which is a vast improvement over bone marrow tests that are routinely given after treatment.

Leukemia Research Funding

Leukemia research is funded through private organizations such as the Leukemia & Lymphoma Society and the federal government. Although the National Institutes of Health allocates funding for childhood and adult leukemias, the agency provides much greater funding for many other diseases and disorders.

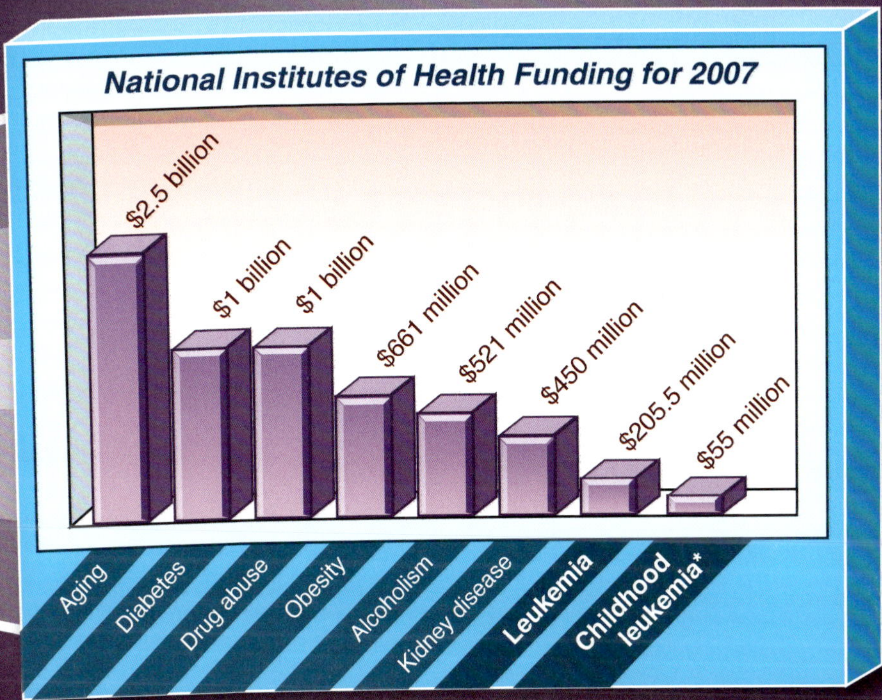

*Funding from the National Cancer Institute, an agency of the NIH.

Sources: National Institutes of Health, "Estimates of Funding for Various Research, Conditions, and Disease Categories," January 15, 2009. http://report.nih.gov; National Cancer Institute, "A Snapshot of Leukemia," September 2008. http://planning.cancer.gov.

- A study released in April 2009 by the National Cancer Institute found that changes in the immune system of those with chronic lymphocytic leukemia can be seen as much as **10 years before the disease is diagnosed**, which could lead scientists to identify the cause and develop improved treatments.

Curing Leukemia with Stem Cells

Of all the treatments that scientists have developed to fight and cure leukemia, stem cell therapies are among the most promising. Stem cells are the master cells of the body from which all other cells are produced. Research has shown that stem cells have amazing potential for curing many diseases, including leukemia. Before a stem cell transplant is performed, the patient is given high doses of chemotherapy and/or radiation to kill cancer cells and make room in the bone marrow for the new stem cells to grow. Bone marrow that has been taken from a healthy donor (or the patient when he or she is in remission) is harvested to remove the stem cells. Then the cells are infused into the patient's bloodstream through an intravenous (IV) drip. The procedure is shown in this illustration.

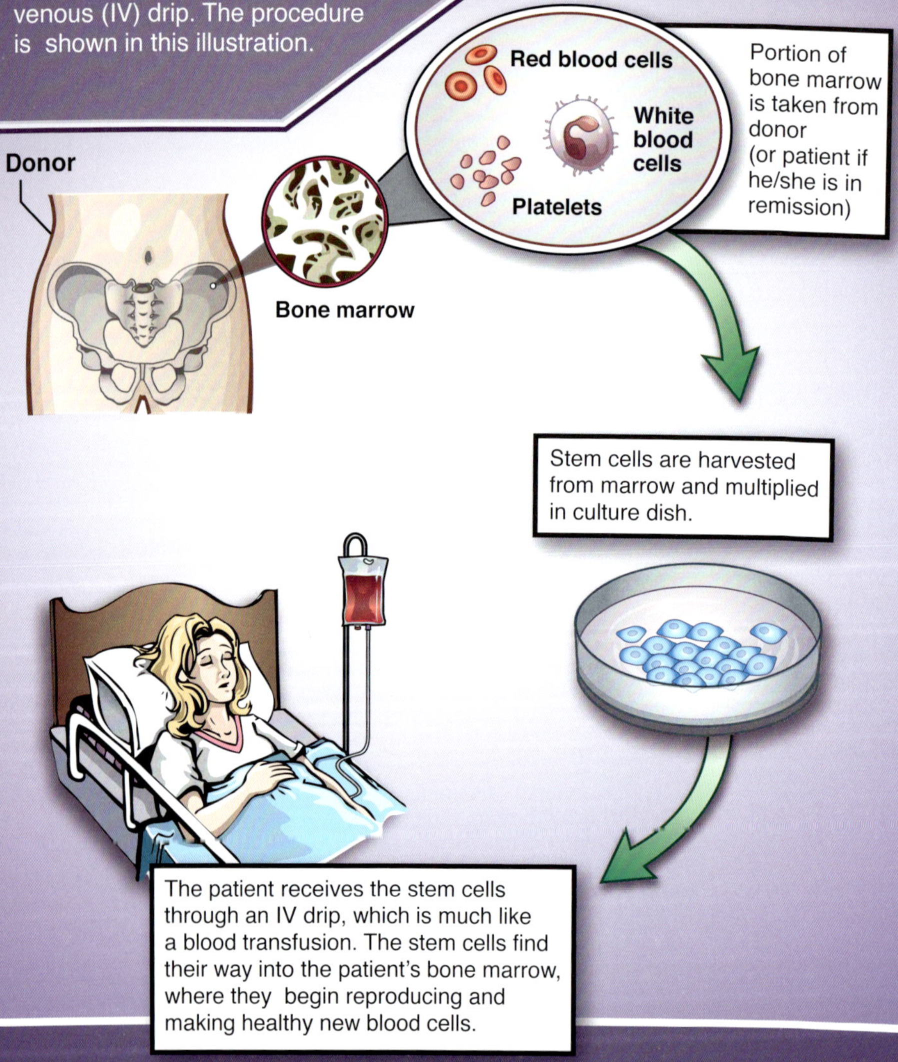

Sources: National Institutes of Health, "Bone Marrow Transplant," MedLine Plus Medical Encyclopedia, October 30, 2008. www.nlm.nih.gov; University of Kansas Medical Center, "Stem Cell Research 101," 2009. www.kumc.edu.

Opinions About Cancer Research Funding

Scientific research has resulted in many amazing accomplishments over the years, including treatments that have significantly improved the chances of survival for people suffering from leukemia and other cancers. Such research is extremely expensive and relies on funding from a variety of sources. During an April 2009 poll by CBS News and the *New York Times*, participants were asked for their opinions about federal spending on cancer research. Most respondents think that progress has been made in finding a cure for cancer, but more than one-third believe that the federal government does not provide adequate funding for cancer research compared with other types of medical research.

Question: What do you think about federal government spending for cancer research compared with federal government spending for other medical research? Do you think the government is spending too much, too little, or about the right amount on cancer research?

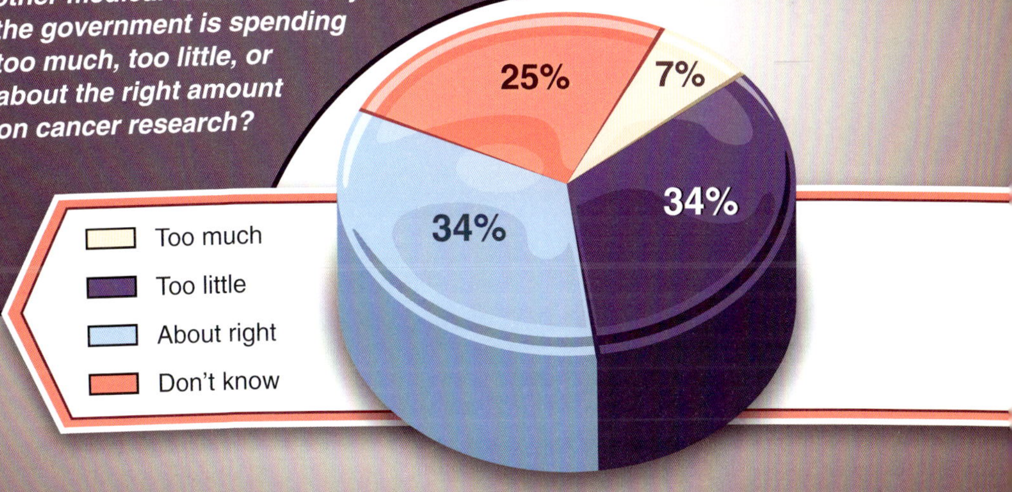

Source: CBS News/*The New York Times*, "Americans' Views on Cancer Research," April 23, 2009. www.cbsnews.com.

- In July 2009 researchers from the Ontario Cancer Institute announced that they had developed the first leukemia therapy that **targets a protein on the surface of cancer stem cells** that drive acute myeloid leukemia, a research breakthrough that is likely to lead to more effective treatments.

Key People and Advocacy Groups

American Association for Cancer Research: An organization whose mission is to prevent and cure cancer through research, education, communication, and collaboration.

American Cancer Society: The American Cancer Society seeks to eliminate cancer as a major health problem by preventing it and saving lives through research, education, advocacy, and service.

John Hughes Bennett: An English physician and pathologist who was credited by the Leukemia Research Fund for being the first person to describe leukemia in 1845.

Alfred Donné: A French physician who published a book in 1844 in which he acknowledged that white blood cells in leukemia patients resembled purulent matter, but upon closer examination were not pus at all.

Leukemia & Lymphoma Society: Through research, education, and patient services, the Leukemia & Lymphoma Society seeks to cure leukemia and other blood cancers and improve the quality of life for patients and their families.

Leukemia Research Foundation: The mission of the Leukemia Research Foundation is to conquer leukemia and other blood cancers by funding research into their causes and cures and to enrich the lives of those touched by these diseases.

National Cancer Institute: An agency of the National Institutes of Health, the National Cancer Institute is the U.S. government's principal federal agency for cancer research and training.

National Children's Leukemia Foundation: This organization's mission is to provide the cure for cancer and other life-threatening diseases throughout the world and to ensure that all persons have access to life-saving medical care.

National Institutes of Health: The National Institutes of Health is the United States' primary agency for conducting and supporting medical research.

St. Jude Children's Research Hospital: A renowned pediatric treatment and research facility located in Memphis, Tennessee, with a Comprehensive Cancer Center that focuses exclusively on leukemia and other cancers that affect children.

E. Donnall Thomas: A New York physician who made medical history in 1956 when he performed the world's first bone marrow transplant on a young patient with leukemia.

Mark Witten and Paul Sheppard: Researchers from the University of Arizona who discovered that the amount of the toxic metal tungsten had quadrupled in Fallon, Nevada, between 1990 and 2002, the same period of time in which 17 children there developed leukemia.

Chronology

1850

1900

1950

1844
French physician Alfred Donné publishes a book entitled *Complimentary Course on Microscopy for Medical Studies* in which he describes patients who died of an unknown disease and whose blood contained excessive amounts of white blood cells.

1845
English physician and pathologist John Hughes Bennett publishes a paper in which he describes two patients who died after their spleens had become enlarged, and he attributes their deaths to "purulent matter" (pus) in their bloodstreams. He names the disease leucocythaemia.

1896
German physicist Wilhelm Roentgen presents a lecture describing his discovery of X-rays—a discovery that eventually leads to radiation treatments that are used on people with leukemia and other cancers.

1901
Wilhelm Roentgen receives the Nobel Prize in Physics for his discovery of X-rays.

1907
The American Association for Cancer Research is founded by a group of 11 physicians and scientists.

1913
The American Society for the Control of Cancer is founded in New York City. The organization's name is later changed to the American Cancer Society.

1947
Scientist and physician Sidney Farber obtains remission in childhood leukemia with a drug known as, aminopterin, which is the first successful chemotherapy treatment for cancer.

1948
After discovering that folic acid stimulates the production of leukemia cells, Boston physician Sidney Farber uses an experimental treatment on a young leukemia patient. A week after giving her a folic acid inhibitor known as aminopterin, the girl dies, but an autopsy shows a vast reduction of cancerous cells in her blood.

1949
After losing their 16-year-old son to leukemia, Rudolph and Antoinette de Villiers of New York City start a fund-raising and education organization in his name, which, after several name changes, eventually becomes the Leukemia & Lymphoma Society.

1950 1980 2010

1955
Scientist Emil J. Freireich and colleagues design the first scientific clinical trial for combination cancer chemotherapy, which leads to a 15 percent cure rate for childhood leukemia by 1962.

1956
New York physician E. Donnall Thomas performs the world's first bone marrow transplant on a young leukemia patient, using marrow from an identical twin.

1963
The average five-year survival rate for someone with leukemia is 14 percent.

1964
British scientists Anthony Epstein and Yvonne Barr identify a virus contained in cells cultured from tumor specimens sent to them by a fellow researcher in Kampala, Uganda. The virus is named the Epstein-Barr virus and is shown to contribute to various forms of cancer.

1965
Scientists James Holland, Emil J. Freireich, and Emil Frei discover that using combination chemotherapy is the most effective way to treat cancer patients, and this approach proves to cure leukemia in many children.

1968
Scientist Donald Pinkel uses high-dose radiation to prevent central nervous system cancer relapses and achieves a 35 percent cure rate for childhood leukemia.

1969
E. Donnall Thomas performs the world's first bone marrow transplant on a patient whose donor was not a twin.

2004
The five-year survival rate for someone with leukemia exceeds 50 percent.

2007
Researchers from Ohio State University's Comprehensive Cancer Center announce that they have discovered the first inherited mutated gene that increases someone's risk for developing chronic lymphocytic leukemia.

2009
The Leukemia & Lymphoma Society forms a partnership with FORMA Therapeutics, a chemistry and biology organization that develops cancer therapies, in order to get new treatments to patients faster.

Related Organizations

American Association for Cancer Research (AACR)

615 Chestnut St., 17th Floor

Philadelphia, PA 19106-4404

phone: (215) 440-9300 • toll free: (866) 423-3965 • fax: (215) 440-9313

e-mail: aacr@aacr.org • Web site: www.aacr.org

The mission of the AACR is to prevent and cure cancer through research, education, communication, and collaboration. Its Web site features an e-newsletter, a "Surviving and Thriving: Life with Cancer" podcast series, fact sheets about leukemia and other cancers, and information about leukemia research.

American Cancer Society

250 Williams St., Suite 600

Atlanta, GA 30303

phone: (404) 320-3333 • toll-free: (800) 227-2345

fax: (404) 982-3677

Web site: www.cancer.org

The American Cancer Society is dedicated to preventing cancer, saving lives, and diminishing suffering from cancer through research, education, advocacy, and service. Its Web site offers cancer facts and figures, statistics, numerous publications on leukemia, and research information.

Cancer Treatment Centers of America

1336 Basswood Rd.

Schaumburg, IL 60173

phone: (847) 342-7400 • toll-free: (800) 615-3055

Web site: www.cancercenter.com

Cancer Treatment Centers of America is committed to helping people overcome cancer. Its Web site features news releases, survivor stories, a monthly newsletter, and information about treatments for leukemia and other forms of cancer.

Children's Cancer Research Fund

7801 E. Bush Lake Rd., Suite 130

Minneapolis, MN 55439-3152

phone: (952) 893-9355 • fax: (952) 893-9366

e-mail: webmaster@childrenscancer.org

Web site: www.childrenscancer.org

Children's Cancer Research Fund is dedicated to finding a cure for childhood cancer by providing funds to the University of Minnesota for research and training relating to the prevention, treatment, and cure of childhood cancer. Its Web site offers news stories, research updates, "stories of hope" about children who have survived leukemia and other cancers, and a "Learning Center" section with articles on various topics.

I'm Too Young for This! Cancer Foundation

40 Worth St., Suite 7F

New York, NY 10013

phone: (516) 526-9371 • toll-free: (877) 735-4673

fax: (646) 861-2565

e-mail: stupidcancer@i2y • Web site: http://i2y.com

Founded in 2007 by young adult cancer survivors, the I'm Too Young for This! Cancer Foundation is considered a global leader in the fight against cancer working exclusively on behalf of survivors under the age of 40 and their care providers. Its Web site, which is tailored specifically toward young people, features news articles, the "Stupid Cancer Blog," newsletters, essays, and a "Support Channels" section that links to forums and chat rooms, as well as many other resources.

Leukemia & Lymphoma Society

1311 Mamaroneck Ave., Suite 310

White Plains, NY 10605

phone: (914) 949-0084 • toll-free: (800) 955-4572

Web site: www.leukemia.org

The Leukemia & Lymphoma Society is dedicated to funding blood cancer research, education, and patient services, and its mission is to cure leukemia and related diseases and to improve the quality of life of patients and their families. Its Web site offers facts and statistics, a comprehensive "Leukemia" page, information about research and clinical trials, and numerous fact sheets.

Leukemia Research Foundation

3520 Lake Ave., Suite 202

Wilmette, IL 60091-1064

phone: (847) 424-0600 • toll-free: (888) 558-5385 • fax: (847) 424-0606

e-mail: info@lrf.org • Web site: www.leukemia-research.org

The mission of the Leukemia Research Foundation is to conquer leukemia and related disorders by funding research into the causes and cures and to enrich the lives of those touched by these diseases. Its Web site features an "About the Diseases" section, frequently asked questions, a glossary, news articles, and links to other leukemia resources.

Mayo Clinic

200 First St. SW

Rochester, MN 55905

phone: (507) 284-2511 • fax: (507) 284-0161

Web site: www.mayoclinic.com

Mayo Clinic is a world-renowned medical practice that is dedicated to the diagnosis and treatment of virtually every type of complex illness. A significant amount of leukemia-related material can be accessed throughout the Web site via its search engine.

National Cancer Institute (NCI)

NCI Public Inquiries Office

6116 Executive Blvd., Room 3036A

Bethesda, MD 20892-8322

phone: (800) 422-6237

Web site: www.cancer.gov

An agency of the National Institutes of Health, the NCI is the federal government's principal agency for cancer research and training. Its Web site features a wealth of information on cancer, including a comprehensive *What You Need to Know About Leukemia* booklet, statistics, research and clinical trials, and news releases.

National Children's Leukemia Foundation (NCLF)

7316 Avenue U

Brooklyn, NY 11234

phone: (718) 251-1222 • toll-free: (800) 448-3467

fax: (718) 251-1444

e-mail: info@leukemiafoundation.org

Web site: www.leukemiafoundation.org

The NCLF's mission is to provide the cure for cancer and other life-threatening diseases throughout the world and to ensure that all persons have access to life-saving medical care. Its Web site features a comprehensive "What Is Cancer?" fact sheet that discusses leukemia and other cancers, a section on martial arts therapy called Ninja Power, information about stem cell research, and a link to medical news.

National Institutes of Health (NIH)

9000 Rockville Pike

Bethesda, Maryland 20892

phone: (301) 496-4000

e-mail: nihinfo@od.nih.gov • Web site: www.nih.gov

The NIH is the United States' primary agency for conducting and supporting medical research. NIH scientists search for ways to improve human health, as well as investigate the causes, treatments, and possible cures for diseases. Its Web site features news releases, articles, archived issues of the NIH *News in Health* newsletter, and statistics, as well as a search engine that links to a wide variety of publications.

St. Jude Children's Research Hospital

262 Danny Thomas Place

Memphis, TN 38105

phone: (901) 595-3300 • toll-free: (800) 238-9100

Web site: www.stjude.org

St. Jude Children's Research Hospital is a renowned pediatric treatment and research facility, and its Comprehensive Cancer Center focuses exclusively on leukemia and other cancers that affect children. The Web site features information about studies of leukemia and other childhood cancers, leukemia fact sheets, and a search engine that produces numerous leukemia publications.

For Further Research

Books

Donna M. Bozzone, *Leukemia*. New York: Chelsea House, 2009.

Maribeth R. Ditmars, *Christopher's Journey: A Remarkable Young Man's Struggle with Leukemia*. Bloomington, IN: iUniverse, 2007.

Zoann Dreyer, *Living with Cancer* (*Teen's Guides*). New York: Facts On File, 2008.

Evan Handler, *It's Only Temporary: The Good News and Bad News of Being Alive*. New York: Riverhead, 2008.

Adrienne Lerner, ed., *Leukemia*. Detroit: Greenhaven, 2009.

Deborah Ludwig, *Rebirth: A Leukemia Survivor's Journal of Healing During Chemotherapy, Bone Marrow Transplant, and Recovery*. Bloomington, IN: Xlibris, 2009.

Jay Shotel and Sue Shotel, *It's Good to Know a Miracle: Dani's Story; One Family's Struggle with Leukemia*. New York: Gordian Knot, 2008.

Louis George Whitehead, *Living Through Leukemia: A Journey to Health*. Bloomington, IN: iUniverse, 2007.

Periodicals

Sarah Baldauf, "After 27 Months of Chemo and Complications, It's Over," *U.S. News & World Report*, June 9, 2008.

Heidi Belden, "Broad Label for New Leukemia Therapy Looks Promising," *Drug Topics*, May 12, 2008.

Avery Comarow, "Embracing Alternative Care: Top Hospitals Put Unorthodox Therapies into Practice," *U.S. News & World Report*, January 21, 2008.

Consumer Health News, "Leukemia Risk from MS Drug May Be Up: But Few Options Require Balancing Dangers and Benefits, Experts Say," April 30, 2009.

Cody Crane, "Defeating a Deadly Disease: One Teen's Quest to Beat Cancer Increases the Chances That Minorities Can Receive a Lifesaving Treatment," *Science World*, January 12, 2009.

Julio Fernandez, "Anti-leukemia Drug Increases Fatigue in Pediatric Patients," *Drug Topics*, February 11, 2008.

Jessica Handler, "I Won't Roll the Biological Dice," *Newsweek*, April 17, 2009.

Nicola Horlick, "Finding Salvation in Hard Work: A Mother's Experience with Losing a Child," *Newsweek International*, September 15, 2008.

Warren Mass, "Seven-Year-Old Helps Children's Hospital," *New American*, February 18, 2008.

Charles Piddock, "Deep Heat: A Leukemia Patient Invents a Potential Cure for the Disease," *Current Science*, a *Weekly Reader* Publication, January 9, 2009.

Nathan Seppa, "New Task: Malaria Drug Might Inhibit Some Cancers," *Science News*, January 5, 2008.

Kirsten Weir, "Cancer Cluster: Why Have So Many Children from Fallon, [Nevada,] Developed Cancer?" *Current Science*, a *Weekly Reader* Publication, February 1, 2008.

Internet Sources

Leukaemia Foundation, "Patients' Stories," 2008. www.leukaemia.org.au/web/aboutdiseases/living_patientsstories.php.

Leukemia & Lymphoma Society, "Leukemia Facts & Statistics," April 30, 2009. www.leukemia-lymphoma.org/all_page.adp?item_id=9346.

M.D. Anderson Cancer Center, "Living with Leukemia," August 20, 2008. www.mdanderson.org/patient-and-cancer-information/cancer-information/cancer-types/leukemia/living-with-leukemia-2008.pdf.

Robin E. Miller, "Childhood Cancer: Leukemia," KidsHealth, June 2007. http://kidshealth.org/parent/medical/cancer/cancer_leukemia.html.

National Cancer Institute, "What You Need to Know About Leukemia," September 2008. www.cancer.gov/cancertopics/wyntk/leukemia.pdf.

National Institutes of Health, "X-Plain Leukemia," April 16, 2008. www.nlm.nih.gov/medlineplus/tutorials/leukemia/oc169103.pdf.

Source Notes

Overview

1. Anonymous, "Kaden's Leukemia Story," Leukemia-Cure, November 13, 2008. www.leukemia-cure.com.
2. American Association for Cancer Research, "Leukemia," June 21, 2008. www.aacr.org.
3. National Institutes of Health, "X-Plain Leukemia," April 16, 2008. www.nlm.nih.gov.
4. Jesse Gonzalez, "Leukemia Survivors: Jesse Gonzalez," Cancer Treatment Centers of America, March 14, 2008. www.cancercenter.com.
5. Quoted in Siteman Cancer Center, "A Patient's Story," 2009. www.siteman.wustl.edu.
6. Nicola Horlick, "Finding Salvation in Hard Work: A Mother's Experience with Losing a Child," *Newsweek International*, September 15, 2008.
7. American Association for Cancer Research, "Leukemia," June 23, 2008. www.aacr.org.
8. Quoted in Mark Henderson, "Twin Girls Lead Scientists to Secret of Childhood Cancer," *Times (London)*, January 18, 2008. www.timesonline.co.uk.
9. Emil J. Freireich, "A Word on Leukemia and Progress from Dr. Emil J.," Accelerate Progress, 2009. http://accelerateprogress.org.

What Is Leukemia?

10. Quoted in Laurent Degos, "John Hughes Bennett, Rudolph Virchow . . . and Alfred Donné: The First Description of Leukemia," *Hematology Journal*, 2001. http://online.haematologica.org.
11. Quoted in Rachael Hartman, "Teen Wins Battle with Leukemia," *Beaumont (TX) Enterprise*, June 22, 2009. www.beaumontenterprise.com.
12. Princeton University WordNet, July 1, 2009. http://wordnet.princeton.edu.
13. Quoted in Joe Fahy, "The Richmond Girls of Cranberry in a Fight for Life Against Rare Leukemia," *Pittsburgh Post-Gazette*, December 24, 2007. www.post-gazette.com.
14. Quoted in Claire Hosmann, "Lifewatch: Stem Cell Cancer Treatment," WECT, December 10, 2008. www.wect.com.
15. Quoted in Cynthia Dermody, "A Brave Battle Against Leukemia and a Mother's Promise," *Reader's Digest*, January 2008. www.rd.com.
16. Quoted in Toya Graham, "Toddler's Comeback: Fighting Leukemia," *Fort Mill (SC) Times*, May 26, 2009. www.fortmilltimes.com.

What Causes Leukemia?

17. American Cancer Society, "Do We Know What Causes Leukemia?" 2009. www.cancer.org.
18. American Cancer Society, "What Are the Risk Factors for Childhood Leukemia?" May 14, 2009. www.cancer.org.
19. Quoted in Aimee Levitt, "When Life Is Short," *St. Louis News*, June 24, 2008. www.riverfronttimes.com.
20. American Cancer Society, "What Are the Risk Factors for Childhood Leukemia?"
21. Craig Steinmaus et al., "Probability Estimates for the Unique Childhood Leukemia Cluster in Fallon, Nevada, and Risks Near Other U.S. Military

Aviation Facilities," *Environmental Health Perspectives*, May 2004. www.pubmedcentral.nih.gov.

22. Quoted in Mari N. Jensen, "Elevated Tungsten Coincides with Nevada Leukemia Cluster, Tree Rings Show," Innovations-Report, February 5, 2007. www.innovations-report.com.
23. Quoted in Agence France-Presse, "Inexplicable Leukemia Cases Rock German Town," Mother Nature Network, July 6, 2009. www.mnn.com.

How Successful Are Leukemia Treatments?

24. Quoted in Anne Hart, "Hart to Heart: Parents, Toddler Battle Leukemia," *Savannah (GA) Morning News*, April 11, 2009. http://savannahnow.com.
25. Donnie Wilemon, "Remission Induction Chemotherapy," Donnie Wilemon's AML Experience (Acute Myelogenous Leukemia), June 30, 2009. www.donniew.com.
26. Quoted in St. Jude Children's Research Hospital, "ALL Curable Without Preventive Cranial Radiation," news release, June 24, 2009. www.stjude.org.
27. Marshall Brain, "How Your Immune System Works," HowStuffWorks, October 30, 2008. http://health.howstuffworks.com.
28. Quoted in Food and Drug Administration, "Living with Leukemia," eNotAlone, 2009. www.enotalone.com.
29. Leukemia & Lymphoma Society, "Leukemia Facts & Statistics," April 30, 2009. www.leukemia-lymphoma.org.
30. Mark LaForce, "Day +396 TEAM BLAKE," July 2, 2009. www.caringbridge.org.

What Are the Prospects for Preventing or Curing Leukemia?

31. Quoted in Leukemia & Lymphoma Society, "Our History," July 10, 2009. www.leukemia.org.
32. Quoted in ScienceDaily, "New Targeted Therapy Finds and Eliminates Deadly Leukemia Stem Cells," July 3, 2009. www.sciencedaily.com.
33. Quoted in Jennifer O'Brien, "Scientists Identify Key Gene That Protects Against Leukemia," University of California–San Francisco news release, April 8, 2009. http://news.ucsf.edu.
34. Medical News Today, "Grape Seed Extract Kills Laboratory Leukemia Cells, Proving Value of Natural Compounds," December 31, 2008. www.medicalnewstoday.com.
35. Quoted in Mark Schrope, "Team Invents First Technique for Producing Promising Anti-leukemia Agent," Scripps Research Institute *News & Views*, May 4, 2009. www.scripps.edu.
36. Quoted in Medical News Today, "Discovery 'Significant Step' in Understanding Leukaemia Drug Resistance, June 9, 2009. www.medicalnewstoday.com.

List of Illustrations

Index

About the Author

Peggy J. Parks holds a bachelor of science degree from Aquinas College in Grand Rapids, Michigan, where she graduated magna cum laude. She has written more than 80 nonfiction educational books for children and young adults, as well as published a cookbook called *Welcome Home: Recipes, Memories, and Traditions from the Heart*. Parks lives in Muskegon, Michigan, a town that she says inspires her writing because of its location on the shores of Lake Michigan.